THE COMPLETE BOOK OF MEN'S HEALTH

ABOUT THE AUTHOR:

Dr Sarah Brewer graduated from Cambridge University as a Natural Scientist in 1980. She went on to study medicine at Cambridge Clinical School, where she qualified as a doctor in 1983.

Although her first love is medicine, her major passion is writing. She is pursuing a career in medical journalism to combine the two.

Dr Brewer is the resident doctor to the *Daily Mirror* and writes regularly for a wide variety of lay and professional magazines.

Her other books include:

The Bluffers' Guide to Sex (Ravette)

The Body Awareness Programme (Bantam)

The Hypochondriac's Dictionary of Ill Health (with Simon Brett; Headline)

Preconceptual Care (Optima)

What Worries Women Most (Piccadilly Press)

THE COMPLETE BOOK OF MEN'S HEALTH

Dr Sarah Brewer

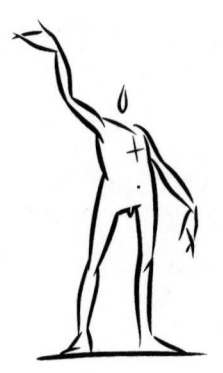

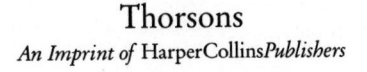

Thorsons
An Imprint of HarperCollins*Publishers*

Thorsons
An Imprint of HarperCollins*Publishers*
77–85 Fulham Palace Road,
Hammersmith, London W6 8JB

The Thorsons website address is: www.Thorsons.com

Published by Thorsons 1995
This edition 1999

10 9 8 7 6 5 4 3 2 1

© Dr Sarah Brewer 1995

Dr Sarah Brewer asserts the moral right to
be identified as the author of this work

A catalogue record for this book
is available from the British Library

ISBN 0 7225 3905 3

Printed in Great Britain by Creative Print and Design (Wales), Ebbw Vale

Dedicated to any man who has ever worried about his health—and to those who start worrying after reading this book.

CONTENTS

PART III: NUTRITION AND LIFESTYLE

LIST OF ILLUSTRATIONS

ACKNOWLEDGEMENTS

WITH THANKS TO:
Richard Marchant: for essential backup
Serafina Clarke: for yet again surpassing her role as agent
Microsoft: for allowing me to throw away my pen
Mark Schroeder: for his computer wizardry
Erwin Ansari: for the loan of his library

Most men know more about a woman's monthly cycle than they do about their own body and its sexual health. A recent survey showed that males are more knowledgeable about breast cancer and pre-menstrual syndrome than about testicular cancer or prostate gland enlargement. This is surprising, considering that:

- 80 per cent of males will eventually need treatment for prostate problems
- prostate cancer is as common as female breast cancer
- testicular cancer is the commonest malignancy in males between the ages of 20 and 40.

Even if a man does recognize he has a health problem, he frequently ignores it in the hope it will go away. Four out of every five males admit to taking too long before seeking medical advice. This is borne out by the fact that, of those people who do not consult their doctor at least once per year, over two thirds are male. Men are four times less likely to consult a doctor about their health worries than women – but are more likely to have an emergency admission to hospital with serious illnesses such as a heart attack or stroke.

One problem is that men are not used to discussing embarrassing subjects, or having intimate investigations performed. This may be a cultural difference, as research shows that German and American males are twice as likely to have had a rectal examination than men in France, and four times more likely to have had one than British males.

Male health desperately needs improving. Men are more likely to die prematurely at any age up to 65 than a woman born in the same year:

- an 18-year-old male has an 80 per cent chance of surviving to the age of 65; an 18-year-old female has an 88 per cent chance of surviving to the age of 65.
- Men have an average life expectancy of 72, compared with 78 for women.

Many of the reasons why males tend to die younger than women are related to differences in diet and lifestyle. Health professionals are now targeting males in an attempt to improve their health. Unfortunately – or perhaps fortunately – there is considerable room for improvement:

- 45 per cent of men are overweight.
- 13 per cent of men are obese – almost double the figure of four years ago.
- 80 per cent of men do not exercise at least three times per week.
- 60 per cent of middle-aged men are totally inactive.
- Twice as many men drink above the recommended safe alcohol maximum than women.
- Seven out of every eight males has at least one risk factor for coronary heart disease and stroke (raised blood pressure, abnormal cholesterol level, smoking, lack of exercise).
- Only 25 per cent of males with high blood pressure have their condition controlled by drugs.
- Men aged 55–74 are more than twice as likely to have had a heart attack or stroke than a woman of the same age.
- 87 per cent of European males never examine their testicles.

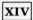

In addition, over the last 50 years the male sperm count has almost halved, probably due to adverse dietary, lifestyle and environmental factors. There are many simple steps a man can take to significantly improve the quality and quantity of his sperm – if only he knew what they were. These steps can make the difference between subfertility and fertility.

This book aims to provide information, dispel the myths and fears and persuade those men who do have a health problem to seek advice sooner rather than later. It also provides tips on how to improve health and diet so that the risk of many common, killer male diseases may be minimized.

How to Use This Book

The Complete Book of Men's Health is divided into chapters that explore the male body and how it works.

Part One of the book looks in depth at the male sexual organs, their function and what can go wrong with them. Part Two looks at conditions that commonly affect men but are not necessarily gender-specific. Part Three considers the positive dietary and lifestyle changes that can be made to improve men's health.

Specific topics can be found by looking at the contents list at the front of the book, or the Index at the back.

If looking up a topic relating to the penis (e.g. priapism – Chapter 1) you may find it more instructive to read the beginning of the chapter first, which describes the structure of the penis and how erections occur.

Similarly, if looking up factors that affect sperm formation (Chapter 4) you may find it more interesting initially to read about how sperm are made (Chapter 3).

Where a topic is related to or covered in more detail elsewhere in the book, a cross-reference (citing the relevant page) is given.

Part One

SEXUAL HEALTH

THE COMPLETE GUIDE TO THE PENIS

THE PENIS

The human penis is the largest of any living primate and, unlike the males of many species (e.g. whale, bear, walrus, cattle, bats, rodents and lower monkeys) has evolved without the need for a strengthening bone. It is an amazing example of bio-engineering, based on three inflatable cylinders of erectile tissue: two larger *corpora cavernosa* (cavernous bodies) on the upper surface and the thinner *corpus spongiosum* (spongy body) running centrally up the underside.

On the upper (dorsal) side of the penis, a dorsal vein drains blood away from the organ; two dorsal arteries, which supply blood to the skin, pulsate where the penis joins the lower abdomen. Several superficial veins are also visible, which drain the skin and glans of the penis, but not the deeper erectile tissues.

The Corpus Spongiosum

The single corpus spongiosum contains the urethra—the tube through which urine flows from the bladder and out. At the tip

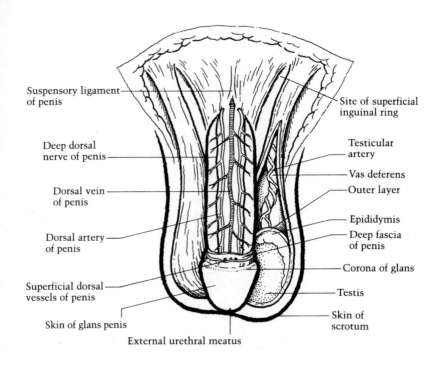

Suspensory ligament of penis

Site of superficial inguinal ring

Deep dorsal nerve of penis

Testicular artery

Vas deferens

Outer layer

Dorsal vein of penis

Dorsal artery of penis

Epididymis

Deep fascia of penis

Corona of glans

Superficial dorsal vessels of penis

Testis

Skin of glans penis

Skin of scrotum

External urethral meatus

Figure 1: The penis and scrotum

of the penis the corpus spongiosum expands to form the bulky *helmet* or glans. At the base, behind the scrotum, the corpus spongiosum thickens again to form the root or bulb of the penis. This is attached to a thick fibrous membrane for stability and is surrounded by a muscle (*bulbospongiosus*) that contracts rhythmically during ejaculation (*see page 53*). The corpus spongiosum also contains erectile tissue that swells in a similar manner to the corpora cavernosa during erection.

The Corpora Cavernosa

The two corpora cavernosa run side by side throughout the penile shaft. Their tips are embedded in the glans penis; at the

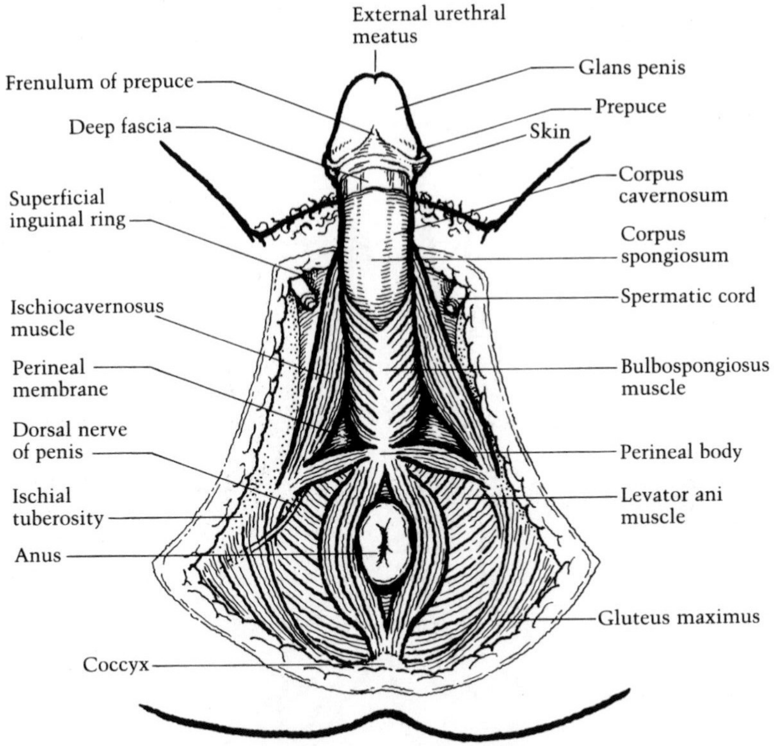

Figure 2: The urogenital triangle and anal triangle

base they flare apart to form two *crura* (legs). The crura are covered by muscle and each one attaches to a bone (*ischium*) on either side of the lower pelvis. This forms an anchorage that allows the penis to stand upright and stable during intercourse. Contraction of these *ischiocavernosus* muscles are also involved in expelling sperm during ejaculation. Further stability comes from a suspensory ligament stretching from the pubic bone to the base of the penis at the front.

The inside of each corpora cavernosa is divided into several cavernous spaces. A deep artery runs through the centre of each corpora cavernosa and its branches supply blood directly into the spongy tissues. When blood supply is normal, these spaces form the equivalent of tiny puddles. When the arteries dilate and the blood supply increases, the spaces rapidly

5

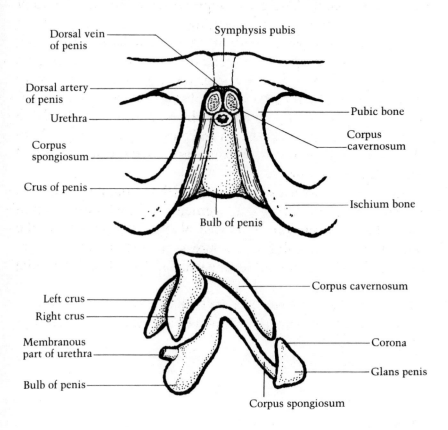

Figure 3: Corpus spongiosum and corpora cavernosa

distend to form the equivalent of giant lakes. This quickly causes rigidity.

Erections

Erections are not under voluntary control but are triggered by emotional, physical and hormonal signals. Testosterone hormone is important but not essential as, albeit rarely, castrated males have experienced erectile activity. Most men, even some who are normally impotent, experience 1–5 erections while asleep. These last approximately 30 minutes each and are often in evidence on waking.

Erection occurs when small arteries at the base of the penis dilate. This is triggered by activity in a set of nerves (the parasympathetic nervous system) which relaxes the tiny muscles within arterial walls, making the arteries open up. Blood rushes into the penis and is shunted into the expandable tissues of the corpora cavernosa and corpus spongiosum. These fill under high pressure to compress outlet veins so blood cannot drain back out again.

The corpora cavernosa act rather like inflatable bungs to prevent urination during engorgement and maintain erection using the fluid tension of trapped blood. They transform the penis from a low-volume, low-pressure system into a large-volume, high-pressure one by increasing the inflow of arterial blood.

In effect, the penis acquires its own hydrostatic skeleton – a method of support also relied upon by lower life forms such as the garden earthworm.

(See orgasm, pages 55–6.)

Penile Size

The size of a man's penis varies less than is popularly believed. The average erect penis measures 16 cm (6.3 in) when measured from tip to base on the upper surface (the side with the wiggly vein). Ninety per cent of all men fall between the extremes of 14.5 (5.6 in) and 17.5 cm (7 in), despite any claims to the contrary!

Size when flaccid is not a reliable indication of size when erect. A flaccid penis ranges from 7.5 cm (3 in) to 15 cm (6 in) depending on room temperature, and generally lengthens by around 5 cm (2 in) when erect. Penises that are short when flaccid tend to lengthen proportionately more than longer ones.

Kinsey, one of the earliest sexologists, had a patient whose penis was only 2.5 cm (1 in) when erect. In a survey carried out by *Forum* in 1970, the smallest penis reported was 12 cm (4.7 in) long. In some medical conditions where the penis fails to develop properly, an erect penis may not exceed 1 cm (0.4 in) in length.

As long as the penis can enter the female partner there is no reason why intercourse and insemination should not occur. There is one argument in favour of a small penis: it is more likely to enter and disengage repeatedly from the vagina during intercourse, which increases clitoral stimulation. Most women say that size bears little relation to satisfactory performance.

An extra long penis is a boast many men make but few can deliver. *Forum* reported one penis that was 24 cm (9.5 in) long, while Kinsey registered one that was 25 cm (10 in) long. The longest authentically recorded penis measured an impressive 30 cm (12 in) when erect, and was 5.5 cm (2.25 in) in diameter. A penis measuring 35 cm (14 in) when erect was described in *Everything You Always Wanted to Know about Sex* by Dr David Reuben, but no source was quoted. It would seem that the longest penises average somewhere between 25 cm and 30 cm.

While a penis with an extra-wide base may improve female sexual pleasure, size is not the great attribute many men believe. A large penis can cause physical pain to a female partner during intercourse either by inducing friction sores or by hitting the ovaries – which are just as sensitive as the male testicles. In some cases, a large penis makes intercourse physically very difficult.

Improving on Nature

There is currently a vogue for surgical enlargement of what nature bestowed. Textured silicone (bioplastique) or fat sucked from the abdominal wall can be introduced just under the penile skin using multiple injections. The corpora cavernosa are not affected.

These procedures aim to increase the weight of the penis by around 30 g and add several centimetres to the width of the penis at the base.

If fat cells are used, the procedure is known as CAPE – Circumferential Autologous Penile Engorgement. Transplanted cells hopefully remain viable and 'take root' within the penile shaft. If the cells die, the fat globules tend to harden leading to an unfortunate side-effect: lumpiness.

An operation perfected in China by (incredibly) a Dr Long, lengthens the penis by up to 50 per cent. The operation takes an hour and is performed under a general anaesthetic. The suspensory ligament attaching the penis to the front of the pubic bone is cut and the root of the penis (40 per cent of which is hidden in the pelvis) is pulled forwards and re-stabilized with stitches. A triangular flap of skin is taken from the pubic hair region and used to cover the newly exposed penile shaft. There are two major after-effects:

1. hair grows on the first 2–3 cm of the penis (but can be removed by electrolysis)
2. the angle of erection decreases from an upright 45 degrees to a flatter 60 degrees. As the penis has been surgically stabilized, however, this change does not interfere with the man's ability to make love.

Sexual activity is banned for three weeks after the operation and erections prevented by drugs. After this, a normal sex life can restart. At present this technique is only available in China, South Africa and most recently in the U.S.

THE FORESKIN

The penis is enclosed by a loose sleeve of thin, hairless skin rich in muscle fibres. This has expansile and contractile properties that allow it to respond to changing penile length during erection.

In uncircumcised males, this sleeve of skin folds over on itself to form the foreskin (*prepuce*). Only 4 per cent are retractile at birth. Most foreskins remain firmly stuck to the glans during the first few years of life and should never be forcibly retracted. The adhesions between the glans and foreskin slowly break down and by the age of three years, 90 per cent of boys' foreskins can slide to and fro over the helmet to some extent. Remnants of the cells attaching the foreskin to the glans may prevent full retraction in up to 60 per cent of nine year olds, but have usually disappeared by the age of 17 years.

After full separation, the mature foreskin remains tethered to the glans on the underside to form a ridge of skin, the *frenulum*, which contains a small artery. The frenulum and glans – especially the corona, or ridge – are usually the most sensitive parts of the penis.

The mature foreskin acts as a cover to protect the glans while flaccid and to keep it in a moist, sensitive state. During erection, the foreskin slips back to clothe the elongating penile shaft.

Smegma

Bacteria, yeasts, stale urine and sloughed skin cells rapidly accumulate under the foreskin to form a white, smelly, cheesy substance known as smegma.

It starts to develop at an early age and is seen in 1 per cent of seven year olds, and 8 per cent of 17 year olds. Smegma that is allowed to build up can cause irritation and soreness. Smegma has also been linked with the development of cancer of the penis, although this is unproven.

Males over the age of seven years who have an intact foreskin should be taught how to retract it and wash underneath regularly, at least once a day – preferably after every urination. This procedure should be done gently and carefully, as forceful retraction, especially if adhesions are still present, can cause injury, scarring and even a phimosis (see below).

After washing under the foreskin it is important to draw it back over the glans so a paraphimosis does not form (see below).

Phimosis

Phimosis is a tightness of the foreskin so that it cannot be drawn back over the widest part of the glans. This may be normal up until the age of two or three years, but in 10 per cent of boys it is still present beyond the age of three. Phimosis is often associated with an excessively long foreskin that contains an abnormal amount of fibrous scar tissue. Sometimes it develops at a late age following a foreskin tear that heals to leave a contraction.

A tight phimosis may cause difficulty in urinating, so that the foreskin balloons when passing water. This can be distressing, especially if urine trapped under the foreskin continues to leak after urination has finished. Even if the foreskin cannot be retracted, easing it back gently while passing water usually helps.

Phimosis in older males causes pain and difficulty with erection, masturbation and love-making. It also predisposes towards tearing of the foreskin, balanitis (*see page 13*) and cancer of the penis. Surgical correction by circumcision is the usual treatment.

Paraphimosis

Paraphimosis is a constriction of the penis behind the glans, due to an extremely tight foreskin. This usually occurs when the tight foreskin is drawn back to expose the glans (e.g. during sexual activity; during catheterization) and is then not subsequently pulled back over. The tight foreskin constricts circulation at the end of the penis and gross swelling of the glans and foreskin results. If this is not treated, the tissues will eventually become gangrenous.

In most cases the foreskin can be massaged back over the glans using an ice-pack to reduce swelling, squeezing the glans to expel excess fluid and applying a lubricating gel. This should not be done as a DIY procedure, but left to the skill of a surgeon. It is painful and often requires an anaesthetic. If manual reduction proves impossible, circumcision is essential. Some surgeons cut the constricting band first and let swelling subside before circumcising. Others perform circumcision straightaway.

Circumcision

During circumcision, the loose sleeve of foreskin which rolls over the glans is surgically excised. This is usually performed for religious reasons, but is also done for aesthetic and for perceived sexual or health benefits.

One American study suggested that hospital admission for urinary tract infection was 11 times more likely in uncircumcised male infants during the first year of life than for circumcised males. This suggests that circumcision improves local hygiene, and requires further investigation.

It is estimated that 90 per cent of American males are circumcised, although decreased popularity of the operation means that 40 per cent of American babies now remain uncircumcised. Around 20,000 circumcisions are performed in England each year.

Circumcision is a fairly simple procedure when performed on newborn babies. A thimble-like object is placed over the tiny glans and the foreskin pulled up over it. A second instrument is then clamped down over the foreskin to cut it off. This is known as the bell–clamp method and is usually performed within the first few weeks of life without anaesthetic. In older males, for whom circumcision is medically indicated, the foreskin is excised and stitched under general anaesthetic.

After circumcision the skin of the glans penis loses its soft, moist texture and becomes darker, toughened and dry. An increased amount of fibrous protein – keratin – is laid down and the glans becomes more like normal skin, losing its mucous membrane characteristics. Some sensitivity may be lost.

The complications of circumcision include:

- excessive bleeding – in up to 10 per cent of cases.
    1 per cent of boys need re-operation to tie off the bleeding point and evacuate clotted blood.
- discomfort – a quarter of older boys find it too uncomfortable to wear underpants for at least a week.
- ulceration and narrowing of the urethral opening at the tip of the penis.

- infection and even blood poisoning (septicaemia) are uncommon in hospital cases, but occasionally occur after ritual circumcision.

Rare side-effects, possible where the circumcision is performed by untrained operators, include:

- the removal of too much skin
- damage to the glans and corpora cavernosa, especially if stitches are placed too deep in older males
- thrombosis of blood vessels, leading to gangrene
- penile amputation.

Foreskin Redevelopment

A Dr Bigelow in the US has perfected a technique that re-develops a circumcised foreskin. This is referred to as 'uncir-cumcising'. The skin covering the end of the penile shaft is gently stretched and encouraged over the glans using a specially shaped plaster (adhesive bandage). This is worn con-tinuously and cut to allow urination.

The skin of the glans quickly becomes less tough, more moist and increasingly sensitive as the new sleeve of skin starts to develop. As the stretched skin covering the penile shaft expands, further tension is required. Either small lead weights or a funnel-shaped expansion device is used during the end stages of foreskin redevelopment. A full foreskin will reform over 2–6 years, depending on how tightly the original operation was performed. Surgical restoration of the foreskin using skin grafts is also possible.

Balanitis

Inflammation of the glans is known as *balanitis*. Inflammation of the foreskin is *posthitis* – if both occur together, the problem is referred to as *balanoposthitis*.

Balanitis causes symptoms of redness, soreness and itching on the end of the penis. This affects 4 per cent of young boys,

13

usually before school age. Older males are also affected, most commonly with the yeast *Candida albicans*, which causes thrush. Little red spots appear and there may be a build-up of yeasty smegma under the foreskin. Screening of the urine is important to exclude sugar diabetes, in which balanitis is often the first sign.

Other causes of balanitis include infection with common skin bacteria, sexually transmissible diseases and chemical irritation.

Balanitis is largely preventable by proper hygiene and frequent washing under the foreskin. In mild cases, simple bathing with salt water (saline) twice a day will cause rapid resolution of symptoms. Stopping using soap may also do the trick. A study among 43 men with mild balanitis showed that by washing the penis with water alone, almost all cases resolved. Soap, by raising the pH balance of the skin, exacerbates inflammation caused by mild infection. Some cases of balanitis are also due to detergent allergy or irritation.

Moderate to severe balanitis due to thrush needs treatment with an anti-fungal cream (e.g. clotrimazole). If the infection is bacterial, antibiotic cream or tablets will quickly solve the problem. If balanitis is severe, with gross swelling of the foreskin, or if it is recurrent, circumcision may be required.

Balanitis xerotica obliterans

Balanitis xerotica obliterans is a common problem that affects the penis in childhood or old age; its cause is not fully understood. The glans or foreskin develops a characteristic white appearance and the skin seems thickened and stiff. This may cause narrowing of the urethral opening (*meatus* – the hole at the tip of the penis) and can interfere with passing water. Circumcision is usually performed to prevent fibrosis, scarring of the foreskin, and phimosis (*see page 10*). Occasionally, the urethral opening needs surgical widening. It is important to have this differentiated from *leukoplakia*, a pre-malignant condition (see below).

Balanitis of Zoon

This is an unusual problem that affects middle-aged and elderly men. It produces shiny, smooth red patches on the glans which may develop into painful, raw, velvety plaques. A biopsy is needed to eliminate the possibility of malignancy (see below) and, if balanitis is present, will reveal that the skin is infiltrated with characteristic immune cells known as plasma cells. The condition can then be treated by circumcision.

Lymphocoele

Occasionally, excessive sexual activity or masturbation results in a raised, whitish weal on the edge of the glans, just beneath the rim. This is due to swelling and blockage of a lymph drainage channel. The only treatment needed is to refrain from sexual activity and let things settle down. As with all lumps however, a diagnosis should be confirmed by a doctor, preferably one in a genito-urinary or special clinic.

Peyronie's Disease

In Peyronie's disease the flaccid penis looks normal but curves dramatically on erection to resemble a banana. When curvature is severe, erection is painful and intercourse impossible.

Peyronie's disease is caused by fibrosis – the progressive replacement of spongy erectile tissue with scar tissue. The fibrotic area does not expand during erection, so the penis curves towards the area of rigidity. Treatment with vitamin E tablets (200 mg per day) or cream is sometimes recommended, as vitamin E helps to maintain tissue elasticity. When erection becomes painful, or intercourse difficult, surgery is essential. Some surgeons excise the fibrosed tissue, while others remove a wedge of tissue on the opposite side to encourage a straight erection. If Peyronie's disease is advanced, the best solution may be to implant a penile prosthesis *(see pages 141–142)*.

15

Priapism

Priapus was the Greek God of fertility, whose phallus weighed as much as the rest of his body. Priapism describes the onset of a prolonged, painful erection unaccompanied by sexual desire, which will not deflate. The shaft of the penis becomes rigidly erect due to swelling of the corpora cavernosa, while the glans and corpus spongiosum remain flaccid.

Priapism is painful and may be triggered by certain drugs, injury or any blood disorder (e.g. leukaemia, sickle cell disease). More often however, it occurs for no apparent reason during sexual activity.

Priapism is a surgical emergency. The penis must be decompressed within four hours, otherwise trapped blood starts to clot and inflammation, scarring and impotence result. Unfortunately, treatment is often delayed as the man is too embarrassed to seek medical help or assumes the erection will just go away on its own.

Emergency deflation (which should only be performed by a doctor) involves inserting a large needle into the corpora cavernosa and aspirating the thickened, trapped blood. This blood will be almost black in colour due to lack of oxygen. Saline irrigation of the spongy tissues is then performed and, in stubborn cases, drugs may be injected. If all else fails, the erection is coaxed away by opening the corpora cavernosa and joining them to the corpus spongiosum. This allows drainage, but will prevent any erectile activity in the future without the use of an implanted penile prosthesis.

Erythroplasia of Queyrat

This condition produces bright red, velvety plaques that are slightly elevated and have a sharply defined edge. It usually affects the glans and tends to be painless. Erythroplasia of Queyrat is a pre-malignant condition, which in some cases develops into a penile cancer if left untreated. If only the fore-skin is affected, treatment is by circumcision. If the glans is also involved, local radiotherapy or the application of power-ful, cytotoxic creams is necessary.

Leukoplakia

Leukoplakia describes an area of white, boggy skin on the glans caused by abnormal proliferation of skin cells. It resembles patches of grey-white paint and is usually painless. A biopsy to examine cells under the microscope will show that they are larger than normal and that the lower layers have been infil-trated by white immune cells (lymphocytes). This condition is also pre-malignant and may develop into a cancer if left untreated. The white patches are therefore removed under anaesthetic.

Cancer of the Penis

Cancer of the penis is a rare cancer of old age and usually occurs in the furrow between the ridge of the glans and the foreskin. It is rarer than usual in males who were circumcised as young boys, and never develops in men who were circum-cised at birth. Cancer of the penis has therefore been linked with retained smegma, perhaps because the bacteria produce cancer-inducing chemicals known as carcinogens.

If you notice any ulceration or a discharge from underneath the foreskin, have this checked as soon as possible. This is especially important if you notice you can no longer pull the foreskin back. It may be tethered by an early growth.

Early diagnosis of penile cancer allows treatment with anti-cancer creams (e.g. 5-fluoro-uracil) or radiotherapy, but more advanced disease requires partial amputation of the penis with all its associated psychological problems. Where possible, the penis is only amputated an inch below the tumour, which usually allows an acceptable cosmetic result. Normal urina-tion, erection and a sex life can then resume.

If the tumour is extensive, total amputation of the penis may be required. The urethral opening is then redirected to open behind the scrotum. The man will have to sit to urinate, but will be able to control his bladder.

In most cases, it is thought that proper foreskin hygiene can prevent cancer of the penis developing. If uncircumcised, always retract your foreskin gently to wash away retained smegma, at least once a day. Ideally, experts suggest this should be done after every urination.

Penile Injury

A tight foreskin commonly tears during intercourse and may cause profuse bleeding. A tear heals only to break down again when intercourse is next attempted. This is remedied by an elective circumcision to prevent recurrence. An alternative procedure is *frenuloplasty*, in which the frenulum is divided crosswise and sewn up lengthwise, thereby lengthening it.

Another common injury is the catching of a long, loose foreskin in a trouser zip. This is also treatable by circumcision, although several cases have been successfully reduced in casualty departments after soaking the affected area in a lubricating oil.

More dramatic injuries to the penis are not uncommon. They can result from seeking sexual gratification with machines such as vacuum cleaners or electric polishers. This practice is dangerous as vacuum cleaners often contain rotating blades that effectively shred the glans.

Loss of concentration as orgasm becomes imminent is a frequent cause of slipping when other machinery is used. A steady trickle of macerated penises and degloved scrotums attend the Accident and Emergency departments of hospitals each year. In one famous case involving an electric shoe-shining belt, the injured man tried to staple his torn scrotum together with an industrial stapler and only later discovered he was missing a testicle.

Non-sexual trauma to the penis may result from industrial injuries, sports injuries and being thrown forwards from a bicycle onto the handlebars. Surgical exploration to assess and repair the damage is almost always needed.

Penile Fracture

It is possible to fracture an erect penis. This usually occurs when a hard thrust misses the vagina and impacts against the woman's pubic bone. One of the corpora cavernosa ruptures and blood leaks into the surrounding tissues. A definite cracking sound is heard followed by severe penile pain, bruising and swelling.

A fractured penis requires surgical exploration to repair the rupture and empty blood clots. The penis is then splinted with wooden spatulas, and erections discouraged using drugs, until the penis is fully healed.

Penile Mutilations

Lorena Bobbit hit the headlines when she cut off her husband's penis with an 8-inch knife. Shortly afterwards, another woman snipped off her husband's testicles with a pair of shears. Both women were acquitted with much publicity, but mutilation of the male penis is not as uncommon as previously believed. Asian women have been indulging in this practice for years: during the 1970s over 100 Thai males lost their penis to their wives' wrath, usually while innocently asleep. In Hong Kong, three cases have occurred over the last decade.

It has also occurred in Britain: in the late 1980s a man was attacked by his girlfriend with a Stanley knife. This caused a severe diagonal slash injury to the penis with virtual amputation. The damage was surgically repaired and, happily, the man has since fathered two children.

More recently, early in 1994 a Chinese woman cut off her husband's pride and joy because a fortune-teller advised it would grow back bigger and better than ever – to restore their fading relationship.

THE URETHRA

The urethra is the tube passing from the bladder to the tip of the penis, through which urine is voided. It is encircled by the prostate gland and runs through the corpus spongiosum on the underside of the penis.

Urethral infections, scarring and congenital abnormalities occur in both sexes, but they are much more common and serious in the male. This is because the male urethra is at least 10 times longer than the female equivalent.

Urethral Stenosis

This uncommon birth defect causes obstructive narrowing of the urethra due to the persistence of a membrane which normally disappears during foetal development. Urine builds up in the bladder and backed-up pressure can cause serious kidney damage.

Mild urethral narrowing is sometimes relieved by passing a slim, rounded metal dilator through the tip of the penis under a local or general anaesthetic. As this usually has to be repeated at regular intervals, many surgeons prefer instead to operate and remove the urethral membrane completely.

In later life, urethral injury or infection, for example with persistent gonorrhoea *(see pages 172–4)*, can result in urethral scarring. This leads to narrowing and sometimes shortening as the scar tissue shrinks. Urethral stricture can make it difficult or painful to pass water and ejaculate, and may even cause

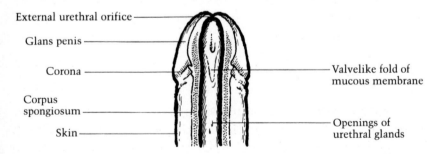

External urethral orifice

Glans penis

Corona

Valvelike fold of mucous membrane

Corpus spongiosum

Openings of urethral glands

Skin

Figure 4: The distal urethra

penile deformity, similar to Peyronie's disease, during erection. If urine builds up behind the stricture, the resulting pressure can damage the kidneys. It also encourages urinary tract infection.

Adult urethral strictures are sometimes correctable by passing a metal dilator through the urethra, as described above. Another technique involves inserting a deflated balloon and inflating it with water to dilate the narrowed area.

If dilatation fails, a cutting instrument (*urethrotome*) can be inserted to trim the scar; occasionally, however, narrowing is so severe that the urethra must be removed and reconstructed using plastic surgery. As any surgery performed on the urethra can in itself result in scar tissue formation, great delicacy and skill are required.

Meatal Stenosis

The hole at the tip of the penis, the meatus, is the narrowest part of the male urethra. Occasionally the meatus is excessively small at birth. This condition is called meatal stenosis and causes back pressure effects on the bladder and kidneys. In later life, infection, surgery or injury may result in scar tissue which contracts to form a meatal stenosis. This is sometimes correctable by dilatation, but usually an operation to widen the meatus is necessary.

Urethral Valves

Some babies are born with folds of mucous membrane within the urethra that form into valves. These valves come together when passing water and cause severe urinary obstruction. They need surgical removal.

Hypospadias

Hypospadias is the commonest congenital defect of the penis, affecting 1 in 300 babies. In this condition the urethral opening is situated on the underside of the penis rather than at the tip and may be anywhere from a few millimetres to several inches from its correct site. Hypospadias is easily missed at birth, as there is often a deceptive pit at the tip of the penis which looks just like the real thing.

There are five degrees of severity. In its mildest form, the meatus opens just on the underside of the glans. In type 2, the urethra opens beneath the glans at the frenulum. In more severe cases, it opens onto the penile shaft (type 3), at the front of the scrotum (type 4), or even at the base of the scrotum near the anus (type 5). The scrotum may be small and the testes undescended, so that the true sex of the child is not immediately apparent.

In all but type 1, hypospadias is associated with a certain amount of abnormal, downward curvature of the penis. This is known as *chordee,* and results in the foreskin only developing to cover the front of the penis.

Type 1 hypospadias needs no treatment. The more severe forms are corrected surgically in a single operation. The penis is straightened to correct any chordee and a new length of urethra fashioned from a tube of foreskin, or occasionally from a bit of bladder lining. This is implanted within the penile shaft so the new urethral opening extends to the tip of the penis. Surgery is usually performed before the age of two years. The child is then able to pass urine normally and to have a successful sex life in later years.

Epispadias

Epispadias is the opposite deformity to hypospadias, with the urethral meatus opening onto the upper side of the penis between the glans and the abdominal wall. The penis may also curve upwards (chordee). In the most severe type, the bladder may open onto the abdominal wall. Fortunately epispadias is rare. Surgical repair is similar to that for hypospadias, but more than one operation is usually needed.

Urethral Blockage

A common cause of attendance at Accident and Emergency departments is urethral blockage from objects inserted into the urethra for sexual pleasure. Collections of pens, biro tops, paperclips and hair grips disappear into the hole and cannot be retracted, often because of their barbs. This practice is not recommended.

Lost foreign bodies cause infection, discharge and difficulty when passing water. They are sometimes visible on X-ray or ultrasound, and can occasionally be retrieved by a surgeon using a long pair of forceps.

Often, a flexible telescope (uroscope) must be inserted under general anaesthesia to find the offending object. Large foreign bodies such as hair grips and pieces of knotted tubing frequently have to be removed by slicing open the area behind the scrotum (perineum) and pulling them out. Urethral scarring is a common and troublesome side-effect.

Acute Urethral Syndrome

Acute urethral syndrome consists of pain and discomfort in the lower abdomen and a frequent urge to pass water. Symptoms are similar to those of a urinary tract infection, but no signs of infection are found and the kidneys and urinary tract seem normal. Acute urethral syndrome may be caused by muscular spasm, especially if the patient is stressed or under emotional pressure. Prostatitis and prostatodynia (*see page 92*) may also be present.

Urethritis

Inflammation or infection of the urethra. See **NSU**, pages *163–6*.

Cancer of the Urethra

Cancer of the male urethra is rare. Any ulceration around the opening (meatus) at the tip of the penis, and any lump noticed in the body of the penis, should be checked as soon as possible.

2

THE MALE REPRODUCTIVE TRACT

THE TESTICLES

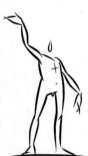

The male gonads are known as the testicles, or testes (singular: testis). They are equivalent to the female ovaries and are responsible for producing sperm and the male sex hormone, testosterone.

The testes are formed within the abdomen early during the development of the male foetus. In response to hormonal triggers, they gradually descend through the abdomen until they reach the pelvis. They then enter a passageway on either side that passes over the pelvic bone – the inguinal canal – and drop down into the scrotal sac. At birth, the testes can usually be felt within the scrotum.

Each mature testis is an oval organ around 4–4.25 cm (1.5–1.6 in) long and 2–2.8 cm (.75–1 in) in diameter. They are divided into 200–400 compartments, each of which contains several highly convoluted seminiferous tubules. These are the 'sperm factories', where millions of sperm are made. The spaces between these seminiferous tubules are filled with nests of cells – the interstitial cells of Leydig – which are where the male sex hormone, testosterone, is made.

Each testis is protected by a tough fibrous capsule, the *tunica*

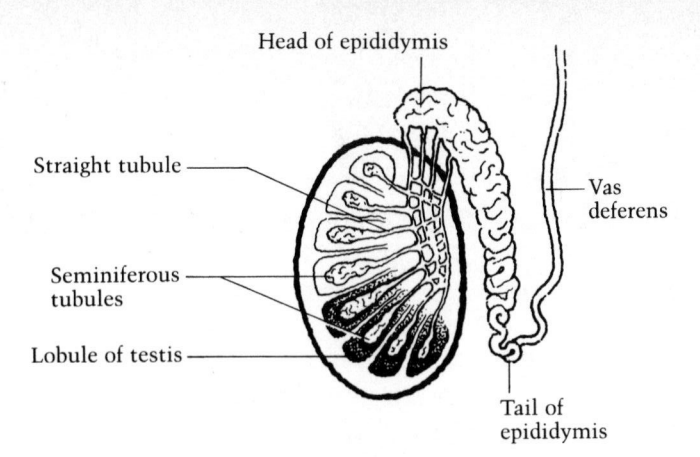

Head of epididymis

Straight tubule

Seminiferous tubules

Lobule of testis

Vas deferens

Tail of epididymis

Figure 5: Epididymis and testis

albuginea, and is suspended in the scrotum at the end of the spermatic cord.

The Epididymis

Both ends of the seminiferous tubules within each testis open into a network of vessels that drain into the epididymis. This is a tightly coiled collecting tube attached to the top of the testis, at the back. If unravelled, an epididymis would measure around 6 m (18 ft) long. The coils of the epididymis are wrapped together to form a head (attached to the testis), a body, and a so-called 'tail'. Sperm that pass through the epididymis are still maturing, and most gain motility while passing through. The epididymis on each side leads into a vas deferens.

The Vas Deferens

Each *vas deferens* is a narrow, muscular tube that acts as a storage unit for mature sperm. During orgasm, it pumps sperm up from the epididymis and out into the penis. The two vas deferens, one on each side, are the tubes that are cut during a vasectomy *(see pages 154–5)*.

Each vas deferens takes a complicated route up through the

25

scrotum, through the inguinal canal and pelvis and passes over a ureter (tube running from each kidney to the bladder) to drop down just behind the bladder. Here, each vas deferens joins with the outflow from a seminal vesicle to form an ejaculatory duct.

Seminal Vesicles

Each of the two seminal vesicles is a coiled, blind sac about 5 cm (2 in) long. They stretch upwards from the prostate gland to lie between the bladder and the rectum.

The seminal vesicles secrete a thick, gelatinous, protein-rich fluid which gives semen its initial clotted characteristic. These secretions are rich in fructose, a sugar which supplies the sperm with most of their energy. Yellow pigments are often present and may be seen in semen as yellow flecks. The seminal vesicles also secrete hormone-like substances (prostaglandins), which have an effect on the female tract. They help the cervix (neck of the womb) to 'pout' slightly so sperm can swim through more easily, and may also trigger wave-like contractions which induce eddy currents and help propel the sperm along.

The Ejaculatory Ducts

There are two ejaculatory ducts, one on each side, behind the neck of the bladder. These form where the vas deferens and seminal vesicle meet on each side. The ejaculatory ducts pass through the single, midline prostate gland to direct semen into the penis, within the prostate gland itself.

Cowper's Glands

Cowper's (bulbourethral) glands lie underneath the prostate gland on either side. They secrete a lubricating fluid into the urethra early on during sexual activity. This may appear at the end of the penis as a glistening drop of slippery mucus. These glands can become inflamed, for example because of sexually transmissible diseases such as Chlamydia and gonorrhoea.

The Spermatic Cord

Each testicle is suspended within the scrotum by a spermatic cord. This structure contains the vas deferens plus several arteries, veins and nerves. It is covered with three layers of tissue (picked up during the descent of the testicle through the abdomen during foetal development) and is sheathed in the cremaster muscle.

Cremasteric Reflex

The cremaster (literally, suspender) muscle is responsible for the cremasteric reflex – the involuntary drawing up of the testicles towards the inguinal canal, for example when it is cold, during the fight-or-flight response to shock (see pages 283–5), or when touched.

Highly retractile testicles are normal in young children, but usually disappear by puberty. It is important that a retracted testicle (normal) is not confused with an undescended testicle (abnormal). These are easily told apart by a surgeon who, having identified the tiny testis at the bottom of the inguinal canal, can gently coax it down into the scrotum with a downward stroking action. Retractile testes are normal and require no treatment.

Sumo wrestlers can train themselves to withdraw their testicles high up towards the abdomen for protection during competition.

Testicular Descent and Undescended Testes

The testicles originally develop within the abdominal cavity of the male embryo, near the kidneys. They become attached to a structure known as the *gubernaculum*, which enlarges to anchor the testes near the groin. As the embryo develops, the testes appear to move downwards through the abdomen – but in fact they stay anchored in the same place. The gubernaculum remains the same size, while the developing embryo and enlarging abdominal cavity differentially grow upwards around it.

Between the 28th and 35th week of pregnancy, the gubernaculum elongates through a passageway at the base of the abdominal cavity (inguinal canal), over the pelvic bone and into the scrotum. The gubernaculum becomes shorter and thicker and acts as a guide, keeping the inguinal passage open as the testis descends. Once the testis is in position in the scrotum, the gubernaculum withers away.

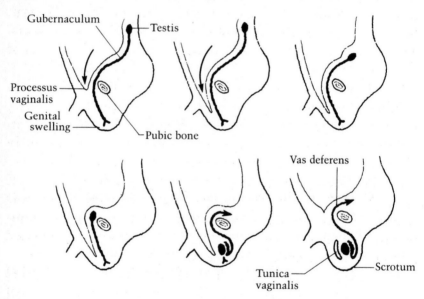

Figure 6: Descent of the testis

It was originally thought that the male hormone, testosterone, was directly responsible for the shortening and migration of the gubernaculum. Now it is known that testosterone masculinizes the genitofemoral nerve, which supplies the groin and scrotum. This triggers the nerve to secrete a protein (calcitonin gene-related peptide) which activates the gubernaculum causing it to contract in rhythmic waves. As a result, each gubernaculum shortens and pulls its attached testicle down.

If the genitofemoral nerve is cut, damaged, or fails to secrete enough of the peptide, the testes fail to descend. In 1 per cent of full-term baby boys, and 10 per cent of premature males, one testis is still within the abdomen or inguinal canal at birth. For babies born under 2 kg (4.4 lb) in weight, the incidence of undescended testicles is 45 per cent.

In a quarter of cases of maldescent, both testes are involved. This is known as *cryptorchidism* (hidden gonads) and is thought to be caused by insufficient testosterone production during foetal life. This in turn fails to stimulate secretion of enough calcitonin gene-related peptide needed to trigger testicular descent. For some reason, the incidence of cryptorchidism has increased by 60 per cent over the last 30 years. This may be related to foetal exposure to weak environmental oestrogens.

In many cases, an undescended testicle descends on its own within a few months of birth, so that by the age of 1 year, only 2 per cent of baby boys are affected. After this time, an undescended testis is unlikely to correct itself spontaneously and surgical intervention is needed.

An undescended testis which is left in the abdomen does not develop normally. It will fail to produce sperm, since this requires a temperature at least 4°C lower than core body temperature. A testis retained in the abdomen is also at increased risk of becoming cancerous *(see page 37)*.

The operation to correct an undescended testis is called *orchidopexy*. This must be carried out in the first few years of life to give the testis the best chance of developing normally. The testis is freed from its position within the inguinal canal (occasionally, it needs to be found within the abdomen) and is brought down into the scrotum. The undescended testis is usually surrounded by a loose sleeve of tissue which pouches down from the membrane lining the abdominal cavity (peritoneum). This pouch is known as a hernial sac and needs to be tied off and cut away to prevent a future hernia *(see page 220)*. The descended testis is then tethered loosely into the scrotal sac with a stitch, so it doesn't shoot back up to its original position.

In most cases, an undescended testicle is slightly smaller than normal. If it is abnormally small and poorly developed, it may have to be removed. This has little effect on future fertility as long as the other testis is normal. An artificial, egg-shaped prosthesis can be inserted into the scrotum to produce a good cosmetic result.

Rarely, undescended testicles are thought to be caused by a hormonal deficiency. Injections of human chorionic gonadotrophin (hCG), a pregnancy hormone secreted by the placenta, sometimes helps to trigger testicular descent and may solve the problem without recourse to operation. This is only done in the rare cases when hormonal deficiency is demonstrated.

Researchers in Australia have patented a treatment that uses calcitonin gene-related peptide to trigger descent of retained testes. The peptide can be injected into the scrotum, implanted under the skin, or absorbed via a skin patch.

Ectopic Testis

An ectopic testis is one that has descended into an abnormal position. Rather than passing through the inguinal canal, it ends up:

- at the base of the penis
- in the abdominal wall
- behind the scrotum
- at the top of the leg.

As a maldescended testis is outside the abdominal cavity and therefore at a lower temperature, it usually develops normally – but is vulnerable to injury. An exploratory operation is needed to find the testis, bring it down and tether it into the correct position (orchidopexy).

Testicular Pain

Testicular pain is called *orchialgia*. The testicles are sensitive structures and even mild injury causes pain. If a direct blow (e.g. kick) is hard, the wall of the testis may tear and vomiting, severe pain and even fainting can occur. An operation may be needed to evacuate blood clots and repair the damage.

Pain and tenderness are often noticed in the testis without a history of trauma and require urgent medical assessment. Torsion of the testis, bacterial infection and testicular cancer (see below) must be ruled out as these need immediate treatment. Another possibility is mumps orchitis (*see page 32*).

Pain may also be felt in the testes from problems elsewhere in the area, such as inflammation of the prostate gland, anal spasm, cystitis, or kidney stones.

Often, no cause will be found for testicular pain and the problem may be due to engorgement with semen or the opposite – too many ejaculations.

Recent studies show that cutting the nerves to the testicles may relieve intractable testicular pain where no cause has been found. On the cases performed so far, all have remained pain free for at least three years.

Testicular Swelling

A swollen testicle should be medically examined as soon as possible. Painless swelling may be due to a hydrocoele, epididymal cyst, spermatocoele, or varicocoele. These are all explained below. A testicular tumour must also be ruled out.

Painful swelling of the scrotum may be caused by testicular torsion, injury and bleeding. When accompanied by a fever, swelling is usually due to infection of the testis (orchitis) or of the testis and epididymis (epididymo-orchitis). Only rarely is a painful swelling due to a tumour, but this important diagnosis must not be missed (*see page 37*).

Mumps Orchitis

Inflammation of a testicle is called orchitis. This is most commonly due to the mumps virus. This occurs in 25–35 per cent of males who contract mumps after puberty. It is sometimes seen without enlargement of the salivary glands in the cheek, but there is usually a history of contact with mumps. Symptoms include swelling and severe pain in the affected testis along with a high temperature. Usually, only one testicle is affected.

If mumps orchitis occurs before puberty, complete recovery follows. If it occurs after puberty, the affected testicle usually shrinks and sperm production tails off. This is due to degenerative changes occurring in the seminiferous tubules.

As mumps orchitis tends to affect only one testicle, there is usually no future problem with fertility. Sperm counts may be lower than normal and the time taken for an affected man's partner to conceive may be slightly longer than normal, but there is usually no cause for concern. Encouraging results were found in a study of 72 young Israeli soldiers who suffered mumps. Of these, 19 had suffered mumps orchitis. Following recovery, some men had more abnormal sperm than expected and their sperm tended to be less active. All sperm samples were considered within the fertile range, however. Interestingly, men who smoke cigarettes and catch mumps are statistically more likely to develop mumps orchitis than are non-smokers.

Treatment of mumps orchitis is with painkillers plus ice-packs to reduce swelling and pain. Symptoms usually subside after four to seven days.

Epididymo-Orchitis

Acute inflammation of a testis and its attached epididymis is called epididymo-orchitis. Symptoms vary from mild swelling and tenderness to a high fever, severe pain, gross swelling and redness of the scrotum with incapacitation. Pain and swelling usually seem worse at the back of the testis. If infection and torsion of the testis cannot be differentiated, an exploratory operation is essential to clinch the diagnosis.

Epididymo-orchitis is caused by bacterial or viral infection spreading from the urinary tract or bowel, or via the blood-stream or vas deferens. The commonest causative organisms in men under the age of 40 are Chlamydia and gonorrhoea *(see pages 163–4 and 172–4)*. In older patients it is often due to the bowel bacterium *Escherischia coli*. In rare cases, epididymo-orchitis is due to infection with tuberculosis (TB).

Treatment is with antibiotics (oral or intravenous, depending on severity), scrotal elevation and rest. Ice-packs may help to reduce swelling. Before the advent of powerful antibiotics, sur-gical drainage of the area was performed, but this is rarely needed nowadays.

If infection has spread from the urinary tract, tests are performed to see if there are any underlying anatomical abnor-malities (e.g. kidney scarring, stones, etc.) that might have triggered the problem.

After an attack of epididymo-orchitis, it may take several months for the swollen testis to return to its normal size. In some cases, the organ will remain abnormally enlarged for life.

Hydrocoele

During development, the membrane lining the abdominal cavity (peritoneum) pouches down into the scrotum as the tes-ticle descends. This closes off to leave an empty remnant in the scrotum (*tunica vaginalis*). In middle age, this remnant often fills with fluid to form a soft, painless swelling in the scrotum. This can grow quite large, to the size of a grapefruit or even a football. In most cases there is no underlying cause, but occasionally a hydrocoele forms as a result of inflamma-tion, infection, injury, or – rarely – an underlying tumour of the testicle on that side.

A doctor tests for a hydrocoele by holding a pen torch next to the scrotal skin. The swelling will light up (trans-illuminate) if it is due to a fluid-filled hydrocoele.

Small hydrocoeles are often left alone. Larger ones may be drained off under local anaesthetic using a needle and syringe. The fluid is usually pale, clear and straw-coloured. Unfortunately, most hydrocoeles tend to reform. To help prevent this, an irritating substance (sclerosant) can be injected into the empty sac after drainage to set up a mild inflammation. This allows the walls of the empty sac to mat together.

Recurrent, large hydrocoeles are treated by surgical excision of the hydrocoele sac. Remnants are then turned inside out, so fluid secreted by the sac walls is absorbed by the scrotum and does not recollect.

In infants, a hydrocoele is usually left until the age of 1 as most seem to disappear spontaneously. After the first year, the hydrocoele is repaired to prevent a future hernia developing *(see page 220)*.

Varicocoele

A varicocoele is literally a collection of varicose veins surrounding a testicle. This is a common condition affecting up to 15 per cent of males, almost exclusively on the left-hand side. This is because the left testicular vein empties vertically into the renal vein a long way up. The varicosities form when the valve system between these two veins fails, so that blood falls backwards under the pull of gravity. The right testicular vein enters directly into the major trunk vein (inferior vena cava) at an oblique angle, further down. Its valves do not have to support the same weight of blood as those in the left testicular vein and are therefore much less likely to fail.

A varicocoele feels like a warm tangle of worms in the scrotum. It can cause an aching discomfort which is relieved by wearing an athletic support, but is often symptomless.

It is traditionally believed that a varicocoele can trigger a fall in sperm count through keeping hot blood pooled within the scrotum rather than draining it away. Any increase in scrotal temperature damps down sperm formation, which ideally needs a temperature of 4–7°C less than core body temperature.

Varicocoeles are therefore said to be linked with 30–40 per cent of cases of male infertility. This belief is now controversial, with many reproductive physiologists claiming that varicocoeles have little effect on male fertility. A varicocoele will usually be surgically excised, however, if the sperm count is compromised in a man wishing to have more children. A trial that followed men up for longer than usual has at last shown a significant long-term outcome. Cumulative pregnancy rates were 30 per cent over a 31-month period for men who had surgical correction of their varicocoele, compared with 18 per cent over a 29-month period for men who kept their varicocoele intact. Varicocoeles are also removed if they ache, but are otherwise left in place.

A new device called a *Varicoscreen* has been developed to (as the name suggests) screen for varicocoeles. This is a heat-sensitive, spectacle-shaped plastic device that is wrapped around the scrotum. As a varicocoele increases the temperature of a testicle, it will turn one side of the Varicoscreen green, violet or blue. A red or brown result on both sides means no varicocoele is present. The test can pick up varicocoeles before they become clinically obvious; doctors in Holland are already using it to screen boys aged 13–15. Around 1 in 50 are found to be affected.

Belgian surgeons have developed a technique that injects a substance similar to super-glue into a varicocoele via a tiny catheter. The glue hardens on contact with blood to seal off the affected vein and causes it to shrink.

Epididymal Cyst

An epididymal cyst is a harmless swelling arising from the epididymis, the coiled collecting tube attached to the back of each testis. Small, pea-sized epididymal cysts are common in men over the age of 40 and do not need treatment. Rarely, they enlarge to the size of a golf ball and beyond, to become uncomfortable or tender. Epididymal cysts are often multiple and may affect both sides. They are filled with a clear, colourless fluid and are usually left in place. If they become troublesome, epididymal cysts are easily removed surgically, usually as a day case procedure. Although epididymal cysts are harmless, any lump arising from the scrotum should be examined by a doctor to make sure it is not a testicular tumour.

Spermatocoele

A spermatocoele is similar to an epididymal cyst, but instead of containing clear fluid it is filled with milky semen and sperm. The two swellings can only be told apart if fluid is drained for examination. Spermatocoeles are harmless and are usually left in place. If they become troublesome, they can be surgically excised.

Torsion of the Testis

As each testis is suspended in the scrotum from the spermatic cord, it is possible for it to twist round on itself. The blood supply to each testis comes from three arteries within this spermatic cord, and by twisting, the blood supply is instantly cut off.

Symptoms include severe scrotal pain (due to lack of oxygen to the testicular tissues), sometimes felt more in the abdomen than in the scrotum. The twisted testis becomes swollen and tender and the scrotum discoloured. Nausea is often present.

Torsion of the testis is most common in adolescent boys around the age of puberty, but can occur at any age. It is more common if a slight anatomical abnormality is present, such as the testis lying upside down in the scrotum (uncommon), or if it lies back to front (common). These make the testis more mobile.

Testicular torsion is a surgical emergency. If the blood supply is not restarted within four hours, the testis will become irreparably damaged and die. If the condition is suspected, an exploratory operation is performed. The scrotum is opened and, if the diagnosis is correct, the testis can easily be un-twisted. If normal blood supply resumes, both testes are anchored into place with small stitches to stop the twisting from occurring again, and the scrotum closed.

If blood flow does not resume, this means the blood supply has clotted off and the testicle is irreparably damaged. It therefore has to be removed (orchidectomy). The remaining testicle is then stitched into place to prevent a future torsion on the other side too. There should be no problem with future fertility as the remaining testicle usually continues making sufficient sperm.

Testicular Cancer

Cancer of a testicle is the commonest malignancy in young males between the ages of 20 to 40 years. It is the third leading cause of death within this age group. Unfortunately, the number of cases is on the increase, having quadrupled in incidence over the last 50 years. In the UK, over 1,000 new cases occur every year, with around 150 deaths.

The disease may have an hereditary component. Research shows that a man whose brother has testicular cancer is 10 times more likely to develop the disease himself than a man with no affected relatives. However, the risk is still small (1 in 450); having an affected brother only raises the risk to 1 in 50. These are good odds if you consider that a woman's lifetime risk of developing breast cancer is 1 in 11.

A male born with an undescended testicle is 36 times more likely to develop testicular cancer than a male born with both testicles in the scrotum. Overall, 10 per cent of cases occur in men who have had a previous operation to bring a testicle down.

If a tumour does develop in these males, it is four times more likely to develop in the testicle that failed to descend than in the testicle that was present in the scrotum at birth. If the undescended testicle is left inside the abdomen, the risks of a tumour developing are even greater.

Recent research has suggested a link between drinking milk

and developing testicular cancer. Questioning of 200 males found that drinking an extra pint of milk per day during adolescence was associated with a 2.5 times increased risk of the disease. No link was found between eating other dairy products, including cheese, which suggests that substances present in milk but not in cheese are involved. The average difference in milk consumption between men with testicular cancer and those without was only a fifth of a pint, so the findings are not conclusive. Environmental oestrogens, including those present in cow's milk, are increasingly implicated in male birth defects, male sterility and cancers of the testes and prostate gland, however.

Examining Your Testes

The only good thing about testicular cancer is that 95 per cent of those affected are readily cured if the cancer is caught early enough. It is therefore essential that all males regularly examine their testicles for abnormal lumps. This is best done in the bath (or shower) when the scrotum is warm and relaxed.

Hold each testicle gently between the thumb and fingertips of both hands. Slowly bring the thumb and fingertips of one hand together while relaxing the fingertips of the other. Alternate this action several times so the testicle glides smoothly between both sets of fingers. This lets you assess the shape and texture of the testis.

Don't press hard, and be careful not to twist the testicle. Each testicle should feel soft and smooth – like a hard-boiled egg without its shell. You should be able to feel the soft epididymis attached at the back. What you are looking for is any lump, swelling, irregularity, abnormal hardness, tenderness, or any change within the body of the testicle itself.

If you notice anything unusual, even if you think it is a hydrocoele or a varicocoele, it is important to have a definitive diagnosis made by your doctor as soon as possible. If you notice blood in your urine or sperm, you should also seek a medical opinion without delay.

Types of Tumour

Ninety-six per cent of all testicular tumours are either semi-nomas (one in three tumours) or teratomas (two in every three tumours). The other 4 per cent are made up of embryonal cell cancers and choriocarcinoma – both of which are rare.

Teratomas tend to affect men aged 20 to 30, with the peak age being 27 years. Seminomas are more common between the ages of 30 and 40, with the peak incidence occurring at age 35.

A seminoma is made up of a single type of cell (spermatocytes, which produce sperm), while a teratoma is made up of several different sorts of cell. It can contain cells similar to those of cartilage, bone, muscle and fat or, occasionally, even teeth or hair.

Eighty per cent of testicular tumours first present as testicular swellings. In 35–40 per cent of cases, men also notice acute pain and tenderness of the testis, similar to that of epididymo-orchitis. This can make diagnosis of the condition difficult. Another 40 per cent of males notice a dull aching, dragging sensation in the scrotum, especially if the testis has swollen significantly. Other signs include general feelings of tiredness, loss of appetite and weight loss. Occasionally, there is abdominal pain, usually if lymph nodes (glands) within the abdomen are affected with secondary spread. Involvement of the lymph system can also cause swelling of the legs due to obstruction of fluid drainage.

Many men date the onset of their symptoms to an injury, but this is thought to be a coincidental effect – the injury drawing attention to the tumour rather than causing it.

Testicular lumps are investigated by ultrasound, which can usually distinguish a malignant lump from a benign one; sometimes a testicular biopsy is performed. The other testicle also needs full investigation, as in 2 per cent of cases tumours are present in both testes.

Blood tests are also done, as four out of five testicular tumours secrete chemicals (alpha-fetoprotein, beta-HCG) which are easily detectable and help to pinpoint the diagnosis.

Other investigations are performed to look for cancer spread. These include special body scans, a dye test of the lymphatic system (lymphangiogram) and liver and bone scans.

When a testicular cancer is diagnosed, the testicle must be removed as soon as possible through a simple scrotal incision. The tumour is then immediately examined under the microscope to confirm the diagnosis.

Testicular tumours are now considered curable. The cure rate for cases caught early in the disease is 95 per cent and likely to increase with the advent of new drugs and treatments. Tumours caught in later stages have an 80–90 per cent cure rate, which is still good.

Unfortunately, occasional tumours prove resistant to drugs. Increased awareness, regular examination of the testicles and early treatment are still a must.

Seminomas are usually curable just by removal of the affected testicle. If there is evidence of spread, chemotherapy (cisplatin, etoposide) is given. Unfortunately, chemotherapy's side-effects include nausea, vomiting and temporary hair loss. New anti-sickness drugs mean that these side-effects are less severe. Seminomas are also very sensitive to X-rays, and radiotherapy to the pelvic lymph nodes is an alternative treatment suitable for some cases after orchidectomy.

If a tumour is diagnosed as a teratoma, chemotherapy is sometimes started right away. If there is no evidence of spread to pelvic lymph nodes, surgery will be the main form of treatment, chemotherapy kept in reserve as another treatment option as necessary.

Providing the other testis is healthy, radiotherapy or chemotherapy do not generally cause infertility in the remaining testis. The sperm count is lowered for up to two years, but this usually improves. Many men opt to have semen samples frozen before treatment and stored for future use in artificial insemination techniques.

THE SCROTUM

The scrotum is the loose pouch of skin that dangles behind the penis. It consists of an outer layer of sparsely haired, wrinkled skin with an inner lining of muscular tissue. Inside the scrotum a thin membrane divides it into two separate compartments, each of which contains a testis.

The scrotal skin is wrinkled and darker than other body skin and often sports a reddish hue. Several conditions affect the area, most of which also occur on hair-bearing skin found elsewhere on the male body.

Infected Hair Follicles

Scrotal hair follicles can become infected just like those on any other patch of skin. Usually, a common skin bacterium called *Staphylococcus aureus* is the cause. A small pustule will develop, which can be frightening in this particular area. If in any doubt of the diagnosis, see your doctor for advice. Antibiotic creams (or tablets) are only occasionally needed. Usually, scrupulous hygiene will allow the condition to resolve.

Boil

Occasionally, an infected hair follicle progresses to form a boil. The groin is a common site due to the warmth, humidity and plentiful skin bacteria present there. A boil starts as a red, painful lump. As it swells, it becomes filled with pus and develops a yellow tip which will eventually burst and drain on its own. Do not try to force the boil by squeezing it – this can spread infection. Consult your doctor to confirm the diagnosis and ask if antibiotics are indicated. These are often given to reduce the risk of epididymo-orchitis (*see page 32*). Doctors sometimes drain a large boil using a sterile needle to remove the pus, and it is always a good idea to have your urine tested for sugar (boils are more common in patients with sugar diabetes).

Sebaceous Cysts

Skin that bears hair is kept soft by the oil (sebum) secreted by sebaceous glands. These glands open into the hair follicles and, if blocked, become distended by their own secretions. Eventually, enough sebum accumulates to form a sebaceous cyst – a smooth, firm nodule in the skin.

The cyst contains a white-yellow cheesy material and some-times has a visible opening onto the skin. The tip of the grease plug may then look dark brown or black (blackhead) due to the presence of the skin pigment, melanin – not dirt as is commonly believed.

All lumps on the scrotum are best checked by a doctor. If the sebaceous cyst is small and causing no problems, it may safely be left alone. Larger cysts may cause friction and are unsightly, so are usually excised under a local anaesthetic.

Sebaceous cysts frequently become infected – particularly in the groin region where bacteria are prevalent. An infected cyst is red, swollen, painful and frequently discharges a foul-smelling pus. This is damped down with antibiotics and then excised to prevent future recurrent infections.

If the cyst wall is removed entirely, the sebaceous cyst should not recur. Often, a small piece of cyst wall is inadver-tently left behind. This continues to secrete sebum and the cyst will then reform.

Fungal Infections

Skin fungal infections are common in areas that are warm and moist. This includes the fold of skin between the scrotal sack and the top of the thigh. The first symptom is often itching, followed by a dry, red rash with a sharply defined edge. If the area is subjected to heavy sweating (e.g., in the obese) the skin may break down to form a raw, sore area that oozes straw-coloured fluid. This hardens to form pale brown crusts. Treatment involves scrupulous hygiene, keeping the area as dry and open to the air as possible, plus anti-fungal powders or creams.

Scrotal Skin Cancer

Cancer of the scrotal skin usually occurs over the age of 50 years. It was the first cancer to be linked to occupation when, in 1775, scrotal cancer was linked with soot exposure in young chimney sweeps. It is now known that chemicals in soot, tar and oil (hydrocarbons) are carcinogenic, meaning that they can trigger tumours. Oily substances left on the hands are absorbed by penile and scrotal skin during handling of the genitals. Men (such as engineers) who work with oily substances should be scrupulous about washing their hands before (as well as after!) going to the toilet. There is also a risk of oil penetrating through the clothes of garage mechanics, machine operators, etc. Where possible, oil-proof clothes/aprons should be worn.

Scrotal cancer causes an ulcer or lump on the skin. This is often painless and not tender. It will start off small and round but will enlarge to form an irregular shape. Eventually, a pus-stained discharge appears, and if the ulcer is hidden in the fold between the scrotum and leg, this may be the first thing noticed. Sometimes lumps in the groin (swollen glands) are the first sign of a problem, though the scrotal lesion will have been present for some time before the cancer spreads to these lymph nodes. The diagnosis is made with a biopsy and, depending on size, the tumour is treated by surgical removal, radiotherapy, cryotherapy (extreme cold) or chemotherapy.

Scrotal Sinuses

Disease of the underlying testis (e.g. a cancer) or epididymis (e.g. long-term infection) can track through the scrotum to form a passageway known as a sinus. This looks like a red hole which leaks pus-stained or straw-coloured fluid. Any lump, ulcer or discharge noticed in the genital area should be checked with a doctor as soon as possible.

3

SPERMATOGENESIS: THE FORMATION OF SPERM

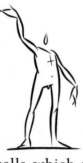

Each testis contains several thousand convoluted *seminiferous tubules*. Sperm are made within these tubules, while testosterone hormone is made between them, from nests of cells called the *interstitial cells of Leydig*.

The seminiferous tubules are lined by small cells known as *spermatogonia*. From puberty onwards, these start to divide to produce the cells which will develop into sperm. Alternating with the spermatogonia are much larger cells, the *Sertoli* cells, which have three important functions:

1. They form a tight barrier between the tubules and other tissues – the blood-testis barrier.
2. They secrete nutrient fluids into the tubules.
3. They act as 'nursery units' for developing sperm.

THE BLOOD-TESTIS BARRIER

The Sertoli cells are tightly connected to each other, to the spermatogonia and to the basement membrane of the seminiferous tubule to form the blood-testis barrier.

Rather like a rubber ground sheet, this interlocking barrier prevents large molecules seeping to and fro between the central space of the seminiferous tubules and surrounding tissues, including the bloodstream.

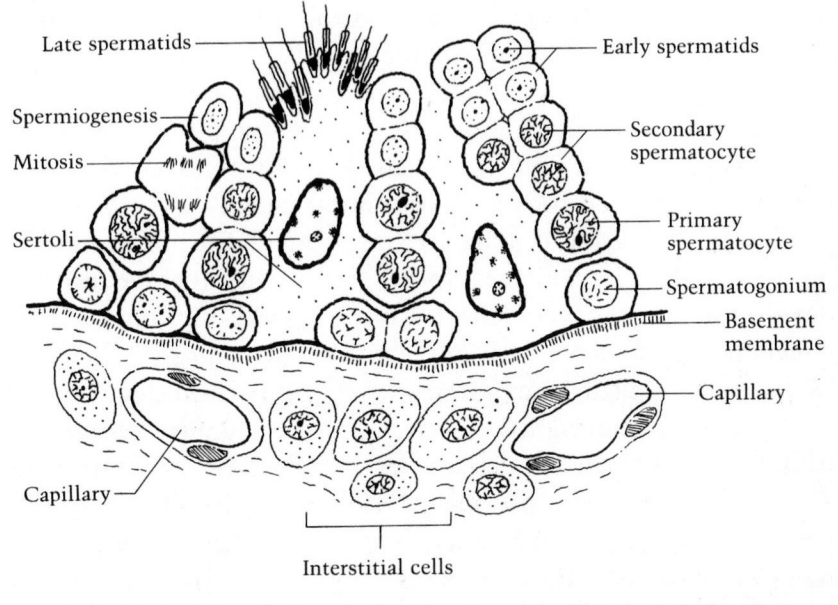

Figure 7: Sertoli cells interlocking to form the blood–testis barrier. Spermatogonia divide so that spermatocytes have to pass up through the blood–testis barrier

At puberty, the presence of follicle stimulating hormone (FSH) and increased levels of testosterone act rather like a turbo charge, boosting the Sertoli cells into action. Testosterone is fat-soluble and can easily diffuse through the Sertoli cell membrane. Once inside, it binds to an androgen receptor and is taken to the cell nucleus where it 'switches on' certain genes.

Sertoli cells start to pump salts and nutrients in different directions across the tubular walls. They also secrete an androgen-binding protein into the tubule which mops up testosterone and keeps it at a high local concentration around the developing sperm.

Due to the secretory actions of the Sertoli cells, fluid found within the tubules is very different from that outside. It is rich in testosterone, potassium and the amino acids, aspartic acid and glutamic acid, which are all needed for sperm development.

The blood-testis barrier is important for maintaining these different concentrations of substances within the tubules. Surprisingly, Sertoli cells can pump fluid into the tubular space (lumen) against quite a high pressure. If a blockage prevents fluid flowing from the tubules into the epididymis, secretion still continues, so the tubules blow up to the point where the blood supply is cut off. This can lead to pressure damage, shrinkage and even the death of tubular cells.

Perhaps the most important function of the blood- testis barrier is that it prevents sperm fragments formed during development from accidentally entering the circulation and triggering the formation of anti- sperm antibodies. It also protects young sperm from attack by blood-borne infections or poisonous molecules. If the barrier is disrupted, for example by injury or vasectomy, so that sperm and blood can mix, the sperm are often misinterpreted as foreign by the immune system. Anti-sperm antibodies are made and this can obviously result in subfertility.

SPERMATOGENESIS

Spermatogenesis is a complex process, involving the constant proliferation of parent cells (spermatogonia) to form the basic stock, the primary spermatocytes. These possess a full set of genes, identical to those in other body cells. The primary spermatocytes then undergo a specialized division (meiosis) in which they split twice to form a generation of cells with a random half set of genes – the spermatids. These develop and mature to produce mature, motile sperm.

Interestingly, when the spermatogonia divide, the resultant cells must pass through the blood-testis barrier as they mature and travel towards the tubular lumen. This seems to occur without disrupting the barrier. Adjacent Sertoli cells form new tight junctions below the moving spermatocytes and spermatids while, at the same time, releasing the connections above.

Meiosis

Each normal body cell contains a set of genes arranged on 46 chromosomes within the nucleus. These chromosomes are arranged in 23 pairs.

The specialized process which splits a spermatocyte with a full set of genes (46 chromosomes) into the spermatids with only a half set of genes (23 chromosomes) is a two-stage process called meiosis.

During the first stage, the chromosomes within the spermatocyte nucleus double up (to 92 chromosomes) and then pair off (Figure 8). The chromosomes exchange random blocks of genes within each pair. This is nature's way of shuffling the gene pool and introducing variation within the offspring. After exchanging genetic material, the paired chromosomes separate and the spermatocytes divide again. Each parent primary spermatocyte has now produced two secondary spermatocytes which contain a different mix of genes, arranged in a different order, on their 46 (23 pairs) of chromosomes.

The second stage of meiosis now starts. The 23 pairs of chromosomes within each nucleus split up, the nuclear membrane disintegrates, and one chromosome from each pair migrates to opposite ends of the cell. The spermatocytes divide again – but this time, each new cell only takes one of each pair of chromosomes. As a result, each new cell, a spermatid, only contains a half set of 23 chromosomes, whereas all other body cells contain 46.

As a result of meiosis, each original primary spermatocyte has divided into four spermatids, each containing only half the genetic material found in the original primary spermatocyte. More importantly, each spermatid contains a unique set of genes – a random half selection from its parent cell. Some spermatids may have a similar selection of genes to other spermatids (accounting for family similarities between future

MECHANISM OF MEIOSIS

In meiosis, a cell in the testis or ovary containing 46 chromosomes divides to form four germ cells (sperm or eggs), each with 23 chromosomes. Germ cells have only half the usual chromosome content because a child can receive only half the genes of each parent.

1 The 46 chromosomes in the original cell form 23 pairs (only 4 of the pairs are shown in this sequence). During meiosis, there is exchange of material between pair members, so that each of the germ cells formed receives a unique mix of the parental genes.

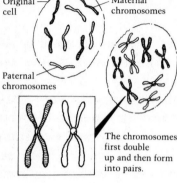

Original cell

Maternal chromosomes

Paternal chromosomes

The chromosomes first double up and then form into pairs.

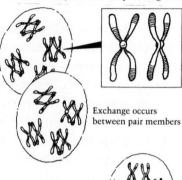

Exchange occurs between pair members

2 After exchange, the cell divides, the two members of each chromosome pair going into separate daughter cells.

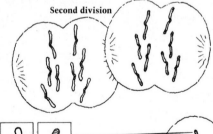

Each cell now has one doubled-up chromosome from each of the pairs.

First division

Second division

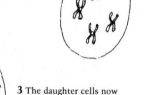

3 The daughter cells now divide into four germ cells. The doubled-up chromosomes are pulled apart so that each germ cell receives a single (nondoubled-up) chromosome from each of the original pairs.

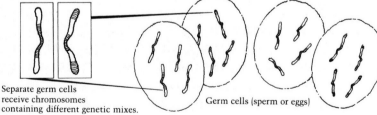

Separate germ cells receive chromosomes containing different genetic mixes.

Germ cells (sperm or eggs)

Figure 8: Meiosis

brothers and sisters), but the chances of any two being identical are virtually zero.

Spermatids

The spermatids look nothing like the sperm they will develop into over the next 70-odd days. They rapidly move towards the nearest Sertoli cell and bury their heads within it, rather like ostriches with their heads in the sand.

Sertoli cells contain a high concentration of a carbohydrate storage compound, glycogen, which supplies energy to the developing sperm. They also secrete a number of hormones, proteins, sugars and other nutrients that help its lodgers to mature.

The spermatids start to grow a tail for forward propulsion, a

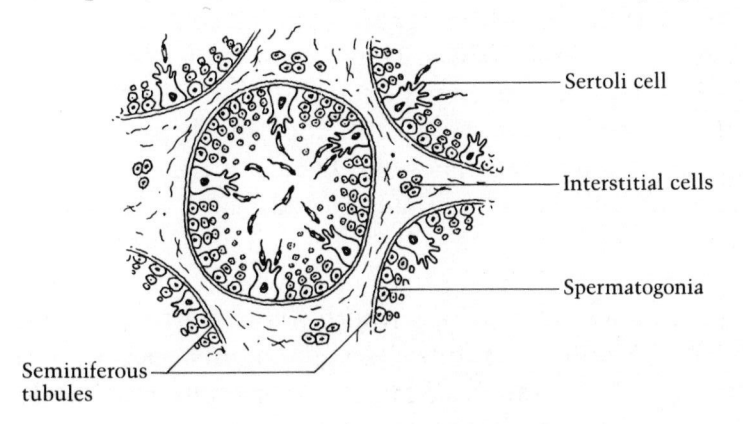

Sertoli cell

Interstitial cells

Spermatogonia

Seminiferous tubules

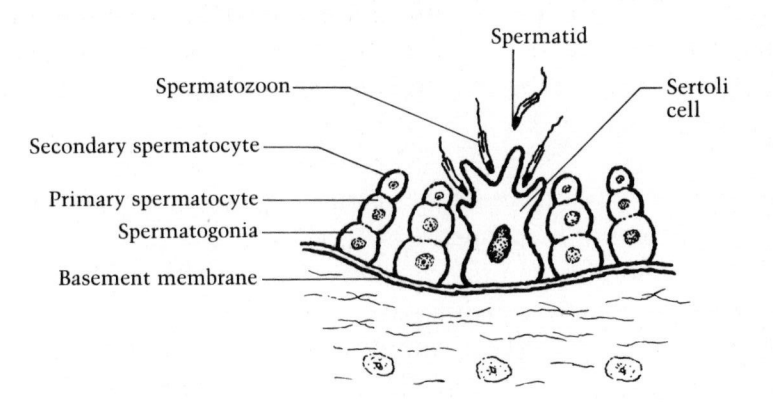

Spermatid

Spermatozoon

Secondary spermatocyte

Primary spermatocyte

Spermatogonia

Basement membrane

Sertoli cell

Figure 9: Spermatogonia, spermatocytes, spermatids and Sertoli Cells

thickened mid-piece full of mitochondria (energy factories – *see page 300*), and a sac of enzymes at their front end (acrosome). These enzymes are necessary for cutting into the egg shell at fertilization. As the tail of each spermatid lengthens, it projects into the central bore of the tubule, waving in the eddy currents rather like tiny hairs.

As the spermatids mature, they are slowly pushed towards the surface of the Sertoli cell. Once their tails are sufficiently developed, the sperm are ejected into the lumen of the seminiferous tubule, although they are not yet fully mobile.

The rate of secretion of fluid into the tubules by the Sertoli cells is so great that a current is set up. This washes unattached sperm through the tubules towards the epididymis. Here, some fluid is reabsorbed so the sperm are concentrated from an initial 50 million sperm per ml on entering the epididymis to around 5,000 million per ml on leaving it.

While passing through the epididymis, proteins are added to the outer membrane of the sperm, they finish maturing and dramatically change in behaviour. On entering the epididymis, sperm are incapable of more than the odd twitch of movement, and if harvested are incapable of fertilizing an egg. After passing through the 6 m (18 ft) of epididymis, however, sperm are fully mobile and capable of both attaching to an egg and penetrating its outer coat. From the epididymis, sperm pass up into the top of the vas deferens where they are stored while completing their development. They are tightly packed together and are moved along by muscular contractions of the vas deferens walls.

Altogether, it takes around 100 days to make a sperm from start to finish:

- 74 days from division of the spermatogonium to the production of a semi-motile sperm
- 20 days for the sperm to traverse the 6-m (18-ft) length of the tortuous epididymis while they gain their motility
- at least six days storage within the vas deferens before ejaculation.

Spermatozoa

Spermatozoa (singular: spermatozoon) are one of the most specialized cells in the body. There are normally between 66 and 100 million sperm per ml of semen, with an average of 300 million sperm per ejaculation. This figure can rise to over 1,000 million spermatozoa in any one ejaculate.

Each sperm measures 0.05 mm (1/500 in) in length and has a so-called 'head', 'neck' and 'tail'.

THE SPERM HEAD

Shaped like a flattened tear drop. The front 'snout' contains a sac of enzymes, called the acrosome. These enzymes are essen-

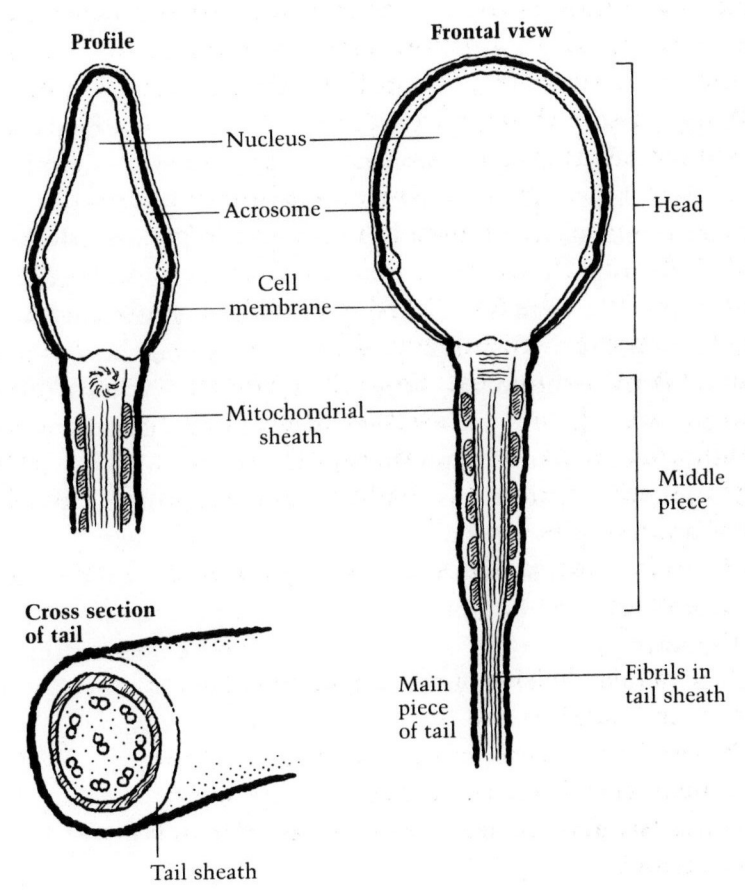

Figure 10: A spermatozoon

tial for fertilization and help the sperm dissolve the coating of an egg to allow penetration.

Behind the acrosome is the cell nucleus, containing a random half set of a man's genetic material (DNA) tightly coiled within 23 chromosomes.

Each sperm possesses a unique set of genetic information which, although it may be similar to the genetic information in another sperm from the same male, will never be exactly the same.

THE NECK

A fibrous area where the middle piece of the sperm tail joins the head. The neck is flexible and allows the head to swing from side to side as part of the swimming movement.

THE TAIL

The sperm tail is made up of 20 long filaments – a central pair surrounded by two rings containing nine fibrils each. At the front end of the tail are a further ring of outer dense fibres and also a protective tail sheath. The tail is divided into three sections: the middle piece, principal piece and end piece. The **middle piece** is the fattest part of the tail. Its extra thickness is due to an additional spiral layer wrapped round the tail which is full of mitochondria – the power units – which provide energy for sperm motility. These use the two sugars, glucose and fructose, as fuel to produce energy.

The **principal piece** consists of the 20 filaments plus the outer dense fibres and tail sheath. At the **end piece**, the dense fibres and the tail sheath peter out until only a thin cell membrane encloses the end piece of the tail. This gradual thinning and tapering of the tail is what produces the sperms' characteristic whiplash-like swimming motion.

FACTS ABOUT SPERM

- Each spermatogonium lining the tubules divides so rapidly that each testicle can produce between 300 and 600 sperm per gram of testis per second.
- On average, sperm are produced at a rate of 1,500 per second per testicle.
- Sperm take 74 days to form and a further 26 days to mature and pass through the epididymis and vas deferens.
- Sperm swim at a rate of 3 mm (⅒ in) per hour.
- A sperm lashes its tail 800 times to swim one cm (⅓ in).
- Sperm must travel through 30–40 cm (10–13 in) of male and female 'plumbing' to reach the Fallopian tube – this is equivalent to swimming more than 100,000 times their own length.
- Sperm reach the Fallopian tubes within 30–60 minutes after ejaculation into the female tract, helped along by eddy currents.
- Sperm normally only survive in the vagina for up to six hours as the acid vaginal secretions are hostile – once in the alkaline mucus of the cervix, however, they can survive for several days.
- The average survival time for a sperm in the female reproductive tract is 3–4 days – live sperm have been found in the female tract 7 days after ejaculation, but whether or not they are capable of fertilization remains unknown.

THE MECHANICS OF SEXUAL REPRODUCTION

Ejaculation

During intercourse, friction between the glans penis and the vaginal walls stimulates the nerve endings of the smooth muscle lining the male reproductive tract. When stimulation reaches a pre-ordained threshold, it triggers ejaculation. (This threshold differs from man to man, a result of inheritance, culture, taboos, training, etc.)

Ejaculation is a nervous reflex controlled by the spinal cord. It occurs in two parts:

1. Emission – in which semen moves through the ejaculatory ducts (running through the prostate gland) and into the central tube of the penis – the urethra
2. Ejaculation proper – in which semen is propelled out of the urethra by contraction of pelvic muscles.

Contraction of muscles in the epididymis and vas deferens propel semen upwards towards the penis. Each vas deferens is the thickness of a pencil, yet the central channel running through it is only 0.25 to 0.33 mm in diameter – the width of a coarse hair. The remaining thickness of the vas is composed of muscle, needed to milk the sperm up from the testes so quickly during ejaculation.

Sperm take a rather complicated route from the testes as a result of the testes descent through the abdomen during foetal development *(see page 27)*. They pass up through the two vas deferens, over and behind the bladder, and into the ejaculatory ducts. From here, they pass into the urethra, where they are joined by secretions from the seminal vesicles and prostate gland.

The muscles surrounding the base of the penis, the bulbosp on- giosus (also called the bulbocavernosus) and the ischiocav- ernosus muscles constrict and help to propel semen through the penis. At the same time, the internal sphincter (valve) that closes off the neck of the bladder constricts, so sperm are directed out towards the tip of the penis, rather than upwards into the bladder. Retrograde ejaculation (where the sperm backtrack up into the bladder so nothing comes out of the end of the penis during ejaculation) is common after prostate oper- ations, in which one of the bladder sphincters is often destroyed.

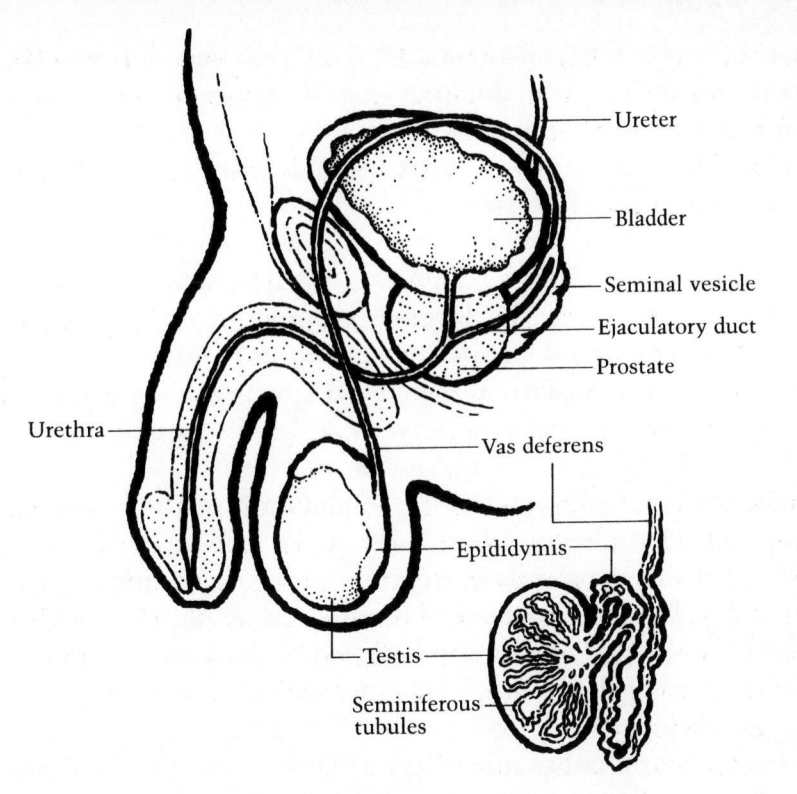

Figure 11: The male reproductive tract. The route that sperm take during ejaculation.

Orgasm

The first stage of orgasm, the excitement phase, occurs when stimuli from a number of sources (psychological, tactile, visual, olfactory, etc.) raise sexual interest and trigger an erection. (For details on erection, *see page 6*.)

During sexual intercourse, increased amounts of the hormone adrenaline and its relative, noradrenaline (a neurotransmitter), are released from the adrenal glands. This increases the heart rate and the amount of blood pumped through the heart with each contraction. Palpitations may be felt and blood pressure rises. Breathing becomes rapid and flushing of the face and chest is common, along with perspiration. The nipples become erect and the scrotal skin thickens and contracts. The testes are reflexly drawn up towards the base of the penis and may

55

increase in volume by as much as 50 per cent due to congestion with blood. The thickness of the penis at the coronal ridge of the glans increases to improve friction, and drops of lubricating fluid from Cowper's glands ooze out of the tip of the penis. These changes all occur during the plateau phase of orgasm, which can last from a few seconds to several minutes, even as long as an hour if sexual intercourse is deliberately prolonged. If the level of stimulation is inadequate, orgasm does not occur and sexual arousal will subside. If stimulation is adequate, the physical effects noted during the plateau phase become more intense and culminate in orgasm.

The orgasmic phase consists of an intensely pleasurable sensation variously described as emanating in the brain, the penis, the testicles or everywhere. It is accompanied in the male by a varying number of major muscle contractions (typically 3–8) followed by several smaller ones. Nerve impulses spread via the pudendal nerves and cause rhythmic, wave-like contractions of the pelvic floor muscles and sometimes of the thigh muscles as well. Contraction of muscles lining the reproductive tract propel sperm up from the testes and out through the penis. Male orgasms usually last from 3–10 seconds, and rarely longer than 15 seconds.

During orgasm, a number of brain chemicals are released: prolactin hormone, phenylethylamine (also found in chocolate) and endorphin. The latter two are addictive, and abstinence may result in cravings and mild depression.

Heart rate and blood pressure peak during orgasm, and hyperventilation is common. The rectal sphincter may contract and involuntary vocalizations occur as pleasurable sensations wash through the body.

After orgasm, a period of resolution follows when heart rate, blood pressure and genital blood flow gradually return to normal. Nerves that trigger relaxation of the muscles lining the reproductive tract come into play, and the arteries supplying blood to the penis close down. Muscle fibres lining the cavernous spaces in the corpus spongiosum and corpora cavernosa also contract, reducing the volume of blood that the spongy tissue can hold. This relieves the pressure on the outlet veins and maximizes venous drainage so that flaccidity soon occurs. The resolution phase occurs rapidly over the space of a few minutes, providing orgasm has occurred. If the plateau phase does not end in orgasm, resolution may take several hours. This results in pelvic congestion and heavy, dragging sensations in the loins, and testes which can be uncomfortable.

After a successful male orgasm, an absolute refractory period is seen, in which further orgasm is impossible. This is probably related to the high levels of adrenaline flowing round the body. Inhibitory centres in the brain may be switched on as well. In young males, the refractory period is short, often only a few minutes, but in most males past middle age it lasts at least 20 minutes, and often longer. Interestingly, a new sexual partner may arouse interest enough to shorten the usual refractory period.

In females, there seems to be no refractory period, so multiple orgasms are possible. Female orgasms lasting up to a minute have also been claimed.

If ejaculation does not occur over a prolonged period, sperm start to build up inside the vas deferens. Some get broken down and reabsorbed while others dribble through the end of the vas deferens into the urethra and wash away unnoticed in the urine. Eventually, nature will take control and sperm past their sell-by date will be discharged via a nocturnal emission (wet dream).

Semen

Semen is made up of a solution of spermatozoa in seminal fluid. This is usually ejaculated in a set order. The first few drops of ejaculate tend to come from Cowper's lubricating glands. The next portion consists of prostatic secretions which are free of sperm and contain substances which give semen its characteristic smell. Then follows the sperm-rich secretions from the two epididymes which make up the middle part of the ejaculate. Finally, the last fraction of the ejaculate consists of the thick, viscous secretions from the seminal vesicle.

This order of ejaculation is not invariable, however, and reflex spasm in different parts of the male tract can result in semen being ejaculated 'out of order'. This doesn't seem to cause a problem, as fractions rapidly mix once inside the female tract.

As a general rule, the volume of ejaculate averages around 2.75 – 3.4 ml after three days' abstinence. The volume varies considerably both within and between individuals. After a prolonged ejaculatory abstinence, semen volume may increase dramatically to as much as 13 ml. Studies show that between 13 and 33 per cent of semen volume is derived from prostatic secretions, 46–80 per cent comes from the seminal vesicles and around 10 per cent from the two epididymes. The ratio of prostatic to seminal secretions remains constant within each individual, regardless of the frequency of sexual activity.

Fresh semen is a thick, milky, turbid, white-yellow fluid with a slight opalescence. It is permeated with sticky, glass-like fibres and contains granules resembling sago or tapioca. Yellow pigments (flavines) derived from the seminal vesicles are often seen as coloured streaks.

Initially, semen is thick and clotted. It almost immediately coagulates due to a reaction between an enzyme from the prostatic secretions (proteinase, or clotting enzyme) acting on a sticky protein within the seminal vesicle secretions. The semen then forms a thick, gelatinous clot. This is thought to be an evolutionary remnant. Semen in many promiscuous lower animals clots to form a cervical plug. This effectively blocks the female cervix and prevents semen from another male impregnating the female.

In humans, other prostatic enzymes immediately start to break down proteins in the seminal clot to their amino acid constituents. Within 5–20 minutes after ejaculation, the semen liquefies again.

More than 32 different chemicals have been isolated from semen, including 24 amino acids, glucose, fructose, citric acid, vitamin C, vitamin B_{12}, sulphur, zinc, potassium, magnesium, calcium, copper and several hormones. After ejaculation, male hormones are broken down by enzymes so the female is not exposed to excessive amounts.

Semen is rich in a number of hormone-like chemicals known as prostaglandins. The name is derived from the prostate gland, where they were first identified, but they are now known to be produced by most body tissues. Those present in semen are mainly secreted by the seminal vesicles.

Prostaglandins have a number of actions and are important in controlling inflammation within the body. Those present in the semen are thought to make the female cervix open and 'pout' so sperm can swim through more easily. It is also possible that they make the female orgasm more intense, thereby triggering strong muscle contractions which help to suck sperm up through the female reproductive tract in eddy currents.

Sperm and the Female Reproductive Tract

Sperm cannot survive for long within the hostile, acid vagina – usually for less than six hours. They need to swim into the protective alkaline cervical mucus to survive. Only 1 per cent manage this, with 99 per cent of semen being flushed from the vagina by leakage.

The cervical mucus is exceptionally sperm-friendly in the middle of the female's menstrual cycle, during her fertile phase. The molecules are then aligned in parallel so sperm can swim through with ease and form a reservoir with the thin, glistening and semi-liquid mucus.

During the first few days after intercourse, a constant stream of sperm swim up from the cervical mucus towards the Fallopian tubes and a possible descending egg. During *in-vitro* fertilization studies, sperm have been found within the Fallopian tubes within 30–60 minutes after ejaculation. Some sperm are found within minutes, but they are often dead – presumably exhausted.

During the second half of the menstrual cycle, and if the woman is using a hormonal method of contraception, cervical mucus is not sperm-friendly. The molecules within are entangled and the mucus is thick, sticky and scant. Sperm become trapped and cannot easily swim through or form a reservoir.

Sperm Capacitation

By the time sperm are ejaculated, most are fully mobile. Mature sperm recovered during ejaculation seem unable to fertilize an egg, however, and if they do so take several hours before this is even attempted. In contrast, sperm aspirated from the uterus or Fallopian tubes seem keen to attempt fertilization immediately they sense an egg.

The longer sperm remain in the female tract, the stickier they become, so they are better able to stick to the outside of the egg. This maturation process is known as *capacitation* and is probably triggered by female secretions. Sperm can also be capacitated by incubation with tissue fluids – a technique which increases the chance of successful artificial insemination. During capacitation, proteins and zinc *(see page 72)* coating the sperm are stripped off, which increases their fertilizing power.

Fertilization

Once a sperm senses an egg, it becomes activated. Three events occur during activation. First, the sac of enzymes at the sperm head (acrosome) swells and opens out to expose the enzymes within. This is known as the acrosome reaction. These enzymes at the sperm head will digest the egg coat and allow the sperm to drill a hole through.

Secondly, sperm tail movements change from a regular, undulating, wave-like motion to a vigorous whiplash motion that propels sperm forwards in jerky lurches. This seems to help penetration of the outer egg shell.

Thirdly, changes occur within the membrane surrounding the sperm head. These changes allow it to stick to the egg membrane and fuse with it, once it has dissolved its way through the outer shell. Fusion of the sperm and egg membranes is essential for the sperm nucleus to pass from the sperm head into the egg during fertilization.

The process of sperm activation needs to occur near the egg, as activation significantly shortens a sperm's lifespan. It is now thought that the egg releases chemicals which attract sperm towards it. Other egg chemicals seem to trigger sperm activation. The sperm- meets-egg scenario is therefore not as reliant on chance as previously thought.

Immediately after one sperm head successfully penetrates the egg cell, a minute electrical charge flashes through the egg membrane, triggering a chain reaction. This immediately hardens the egg membrane, so that no further sperm can stick to it or dissolve their way through.

Altogether, the time taken for a sperm to stick to the outer egg shell, penetrate and trigger the hardening reaction of the inner egg membrane is around 10–20 minutes. Once a sperm successfully fertilizes an egg, it loses its tail, which remains outside the egg shell. The sperm nucleus then oozes from the sperm head into the egg cell and eventually fuses with the egg nucleus. A new individual is now on the long road to implantation and development. It is not until the fertilized egg has successfully implanted in the womb lining and started to create a placenta, however, that pregnancy can be said to have started.

Sperm and Gender of Offspring

When the number of chromosomes within each primary spermatocyte is split up during meiosis (*see page 47*), so that the spermatids only receive half the usual number of chromosomes (23 instead of 46), one of the chromosome pairs that gets split up is unequal. This pair, known as the sex pair, consists of a fat X (female) chromosome and a smaller Y (male) chromosome. As a result of being split up, half a man's sperm will possess a Y-sex chromosome (but no X) and the other half will contain an X chromosome (but no Y).

In females, the sex pair is equal and consists of two X chromosomes. During meiosis in the female, all eggs therefore end up with one X chromosome each.

The Y chromosome provides all the genetic information needed for the development of male sexual characteristics. Without any input from a Y chromosome, a foetus will develop into a female. Therefore, if a sperm containing an X chromosome fertilizes an egg, the resultant offspring will possess an XX-sex pair and will develop into a female. If the egg is fertilized by a sperm containing a Y chromosome, the offspring will possess an XY-sex pair and will develop into a male.

It is always the sperm that dictate the sex of the offspring, not the egg.

Sperm containing the fatter X chromosome are slightly heavier and swim more slowly than sperm containing a Y chromosome. As the Y chromosome is comparatively light, Y sperm can swim faster. This small but significant difference between the X and Y sperm accounts for the fact that roughly 105 boys are born for every 100 girls.

Scientific methods designed to separate sperm into X and Y fractions use this difference in weight and speed. Sperm can be filtered through a test-tube containing a viscous solution of human albumin protein. The lighter and smaller male sperm tend to sink to the bottom of the tube more quickly than the larger, heavier female sperm. Fractions rich in X or Y sperm can then be separated out and used during artificial insemination to reduce the risk of sex-linked disorders in offspring, for example. The ethics of using these fractions to determine the sex of a child for aesthetic, family balancing purposes is still in question.

Newer methods of sperm separation involve labelling them with a fluorescent dye. This process is known as FISH – *Fluorescence In Situ Hybridization*. Semen is then agitated to break it up into droplets, each one of which contains a single sperm. Drops containing the larger female sperm glow more brightly than drops containing a male sperm. Each drop is then electrically charged, with male sperm made positive and female sperm negative, and separated out using electrically charged plates. This method of sperm enrichment can produce samples containing 85 per cent female X sperm and 75 per cent male Y sperm, compared with the more usually 50:50 per cent mix.

At present this technique is only licensed for medical use – for example to reduce the risk of having a child with an hereditary, sex-linked disorder such as Muscular Dystrophy which affects only boys – and not for cosmetic (social) reasons.

Interestingly, it seems that divers are more likely to father daughters than sons. It was recently found that hyperbaric chambers significantly lower blood testosterone levels, and this seems to favour the female X sperm. Studies among Australian abalone divers and Swedish navy divers do show a preponderance of female offspring.

4

FACTORS THAT AFFECT SPERMATOGENESIS

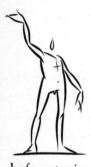

Sperm are easily damaged and need a carefully controlled environment to develop normally. Any factor that has an adverse effect on spermatogenesis will lower the sperm count and significantly affect fertility.

There are many simple things a man can do to optimize the quality and quantity of his sperm. This is particularly important in the six months before trying to conceive a child.

It takes around 100 days to make a sperm from start to finish:

- 74 days division and growth within the testis
- 20 days to pass through the epididymis
- 6 days travelling through the vas deferens before ejaculation.

That's 100 days in which the sperm are vulnerable to many dietary and environmental factors.

TEMPERATURE AND SPERM

A low ambient temperature is essential for normal spermatogenesis. Testicular temperature needs to be from 4–7°C cooler than core body temperature. This is why the testes are designed to drop out of the abdomen into the scrotal sac. Three mechanisms keep the scrotum cooler than the rest of the body:

1. scrotal skin is thin, so the testes easily lose heat into the surrounding environment
2. air circulating around the scrotum can cool the skin
3. the arteries bringing blood into the scrotum run alongside the veins taking blood away to form a sophisticated heat-exchange mechanism. Rather like a hot and cold water pipe running together, the hot arterial blood (coming from the abdomen) loses heat to the cooler venous blood (coming away from the testes), so blood is already partly cooled before entering the scrotum.

Even if the testes heat up by as little as 2°C, sperm formation is adversely affected. Sperm count will drop, the number of normal sperm will fall and the number of abnormal sperm will increase.

Semen quality is naturally lower in summer compared with winter. Although semen volume does not change significantly, the total sperm counts per ejaculation in 131 volunteers fell from 320 million in winter to 250 million during July and August. This is probably a temperature effect.

Even taking a hot bath (43–45°C/110–115°F) for half an hour per day can significantly lower sperm counts – as can wearing tight underpants or athletic scrotal supports. This was shown in a recent experiment where the fit of a man's underwear and its effect on spermatogenesis was investigated.

Two unmarried males in their middle thirties wore tight, bikini-type briefs that fitted snugly against the scrotum for three months. They then changed to loose boxer shorts that extended 14 cm/5.5 in beyond the scrotum for the next three months. This tight–loose sequence was repeated once more, so that each man was investigated for one year.

Their semen was analysed regularly and showed that sperm count and sperm motility gradually declined during the periods when the men were wearing tight underpants, and gradually

65

increased when they wore loose boxer shorts. Changes in sperm count and sperm motility were noticeable within two weeks of changing over to each new set of underwear.

Variable	First male			Second male		
	Tight	Loose	% Change	Tight	Loose	% Change
Total sperm/ ejaculation (millions)	242	301	+20	411	475	+13
Sperm density (millions/ml)	77	86	+10	148	177	+16
Total motile (millions)	193	239	+21	291	343	+15
Volume (ml)	3.1	3.5	+12	2.5	2.7	+7

Source: Sanger & Friman 1990. *Reproductive Toxicology*. Vol. 4, pp. 229–232.

Although sperm counts stayed well within fertile levels during this experiment, it is possible that the type of underwear chosen by a man with a low sperm count might make the difference between fertility and subfertility. Temperature effects are probably most important, but electrostatic electricity plays a role too.

Electrostatic Electricity and Sperm

Tight underwear containing man-made fibres (e.g. polyester) generates electrostatic electricity from friction between the scrotal skin and the synthetic material. These create an electrostatic field across the scrotum, with the skin covering the lower scrotum acquiring a positive charge and the skin covering the upper scrotum acquiring a negative charge. The testes lie between these two electrical poles, and spermatogenesis is adversely affected.

Several studies have looked at the electrostatic potentials generated across the scrotum from different materials. Men

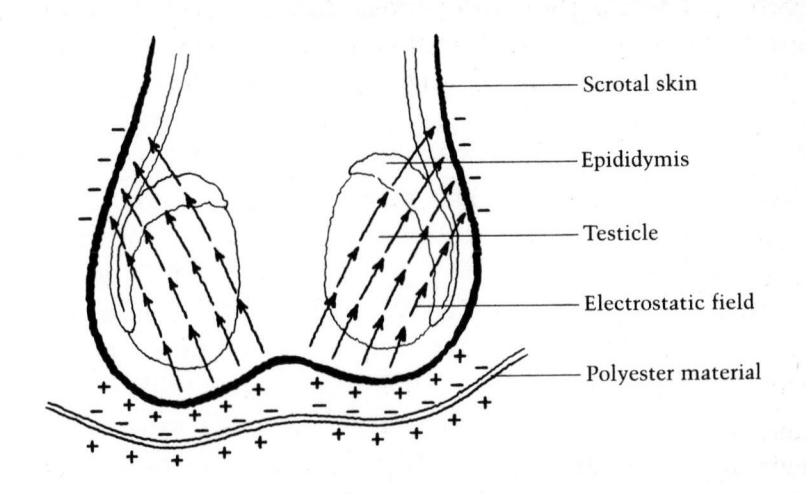

Figure 12: Electrostatic field across scrotum

who wear underpants made from 100 per cent polyester generate the greatest electrostatic fields around their testes. Men wearing 50:50 per cent polyester:cotton mix underpants generate a field that is half as strong, while men wearing 100 per cent cotton pants remain free of any significant electrostatic potential. When volunteer males wore a particular type of underpants for 18 months:

- 4 out of 11 men wearing polyester underwear showed evidence of a significant reduction in sperm count plus testicular degeneration by the 14th month. These changes were reversible once the pants were discarded.
- only 1 out of 11 men wearing polyester-cotton mix underwear showed a lowered sperm count after 16 months. This change was also reversible.
- None of the 11 men wearing pure cotton underpants showed any significant change in sperm quality or quantity.

Investigation showed that these changes were directly related to the electrostatic fields generated, and no significant changes in testicular temperature or blood hormone levels were found.

Temperature and Electrostatic Forces Combined

Egyptian doctors have designed a male method of contraception based on the combined effects of raised scrotal temperature and electrostatic electricity.

A polyester scrotal sling – nicknamed the Jockstrap – was tailor-made to hug the testicles closely while allowing the penis to poke through. The sling was attached to a waist belt designed to pull the testicles up close to the abdomen. This automatically raised testicular temperature due to the effects of increased body warmth. Fourteen volunteer males wore the sling day and night for a year, only changing it when soiled.

During the experiment, sperm counts of all 14 volunteers dropped to an amazing zero, and remained at zero after wearing the sling for an average of 140 days. Their testicles decreased in size from an average of 22.2 ml to 18.6 ml and the volume of semen they produced fell significantly. Biopsies of the testicles showed that after wearing the sling for 6 months, there was degeneration and loss of some of the germ cells lining the seminiferous tubules.

At the end of the 12-month experiment, the slings were discarded and the men's sperm counts slowly climbed back up to their previously normal levels within an average of 157 days.

These experiments show the fertility dangers of wearing tight, polyester bikini-style briefs or athletic supports for prolonged periods of time.

As there may be a link between overheated testes, testicular degeneration and the eventual development of testicular cancer (as has been noted in undescended testicles – *see page 37*), it might be sensible for all males to wear loose, boxer style underpants made from 100 per cent cotton rather then bikini-style briefs made from artificial fibres.

FREE RADICALS AND SPERM

Researchers estimate that 40 per cent of sperm damage is due to collision with molecular fragments known as free radicals *(see Chapter 21).* Cells are most vulnerable to free radical damage during division, when the normal gene repair mechanisms are switched off. As it takes around 380 cell divisions to produce a sperm, the spermatocytes and spermatogonia within the testicular tubules are constantly dividing. This makes them sitting ducks for free radical attack. Damage to the DNA at this time can result in genetic material being wrongly copied so that mutations arise. Sperm may contain a lethal genetic defect and die, or they may develop structural abnormalities such as two heads or two tails, lack an acrosome, or be incapable of forward propulsion. If a high percentage of sperm are affected, this can result in subfertility.

Sperm may, however, acquire only a minor genetic defect as a result of free radical attack. This may even be passed on to the future offspring if fertilization is successful, to produce problems such as an increased risk of childhood cancer. This has already been noticed among the children of men who smoke *(see page 280).*

There are several ways in which a man can protect himself against free radical attack. This is important for every man, not just those hoping to father a child. Free radicals are now known to be linked with coronary heart disease and cancer. By mopping up and neutralizing the free radicals, a man can increase the quality of his sperm, reduce his risk of coronary heart disease and significantly reduce his risk of cancer *(see pages 190 and 205–6).*

ANTIOXIDANTS AND SPERM

Vitamin C and Sperm

Dietary antioxidants are our main protection against free radical attack. Vitamin C is a water-soluble antioxidant that is actively secreted into semen to reach levels eight times higher than those found in the bloodstream.

Smoking generates massive amounts of free radicals, so

smokers are especially vulnerable to sperm damage. They need at least twice as much dietary vitamin C as non-smokers. Men who smoke 20 or more cigarettes per day have blood vitamin C levels that are up to 40 per cent lower than non-smokers. They also have sperm counts that are 17 per cent lower, reduced sperm motility and a greater percentage of abnormal sperm.

The amount of sperm damage due to free radical attack in smokers has been assessed by measuring levels of a gene breakdown product in the semen. Smoking males were given a diet containing 250 mg vitamin C per day and their semen analysed. Their intake of vitamin C was then drastically reduced to only 5 mg per day. The level of the chemical resulting from DNA damage promptly doubled. It was not until intakes of vitamin C rose to 250 mg per day that the protective antioxidant effect returned.

This would indicate that a dietary intake of 250 mg vitamin C per day (the equivalent of four large oranges or kiwi fruit) is a good starting point for men wanting to protect their sperm from free radical attack.

It has been shown that smokers taking 200 mg vitamin C per day can improve their sperm counts by as much as 24 per cent, sperm motility by up to 18 per cent and the number of sperm still alive 24 hours after ejaculation by 23 per cent. Improvement seems to start within a week of increasing vitamin C intake.

Smokers taking massive doses of 1,000 mg vitamin C per day have been found to improve their sperm count by up to 34 per cent, sperm motility by 5 per cent and viability by 34 per cent. Sperm are also less likely to clump together, which is the other way in which vitamin C helps to improve sperm quality.

Semen contains a protein–vitamin E complex called non-specific sperm agglutinin (NSSA). NSSA exists in two forms, an oxidized form which can't bind to sperm, and an unoxidized (reduced) form which binds to sperm to act as a 'non-stick' coating. This prevents sperm clumping together and increases sperm motility.

When NSSA is oxidized and can't bind to sperm, the sperm

stick to each other and clump together instead. This brings them to an instant halt and, if 20 per cent or more of sperm are clumped, subfertility occurs.

Vitamin C has an antioxidant effect on NSSA to keep it in its reduced form so it can bind to sperm and prevent them sticking together.

Studies show that men who are subfertile because of sperm clumping can be helped by vitamin C. Supplements of 500 mg vitamin C taken twice a day can reduce sperm clumping from 37 per cent to 14 per cent after just one week. After four weeks, sperm clumping can be reduced to as little as 11 per cent. Research shows that the overall quality of sperm – including numbers of normal sperm present, motility and lifespan – is also improved.

If taking vitamin C supplements, it is best to take other antioxidants such as vitamin E, betacarotene and zinc as well. They all work together to produce a synergistic effect.

Vitamin E and Sperm

Vitamin E is a fat-soluble antioxidant vitamin. It can penetrate cell membranes and body fats to protect them against oxidizing free radical attacks (see page 359).

High-dose vitamin E has been tested as a treatment for subfertility in men. By mopping up superoxide free radicals, doses as high as 600 mg vitamin E per day have shown a significant benefit on sperm numbers. This leaves vitamin E in an inactive form which is rapidly reactivated by vitamin C. It is therefore important for men to obtain adequate dietary supplies of both vitamins.

Vitamin E is a component of the non-specific sperm agglutinin (NSSA) and, together with vitamin C, plays a role in preventing sperm clumping and promoting motility. It also has a beneficial effect on the flexibility of sperm cell walls.

Supplements containing up to 100 mg of vitamin E are useful for general sperm health. In subfertility, doses up to 600 mg may be suggested by an andrologist. Vitamin E is non-toxic and seems safe at doses of 1,000 mg per day or more.

Betacarotene and Sperm

Betacarotene is a fat-soluble antioxidant which is likely to protect sperm from free radical attack in a similar way to vitamins C and E.

Betacarotene is also a provitamin – it is converted into vitamin A when stores are low. As too much vitamin A is poisonous, ensuring an adequate intake of betacarotene is the safest way to maintain an optimal supply.

Vitamin A is thought to be important for sperm maturation as they pass through the epididymis. Vitamin A can bind to sperm at special receptor sites and seems to enter the egg at fertilization. Sperm vitamin A may be important during the early stages of foetal development.

Zinc and Sperm

Zinc is an antioxidant mineral that is also important in protecting sperm against free radical attack. Semen is rich in zinc, with each ejaculate containing 5 mg – one third of the recommended daily nutrient intake. This would imply that it plays an important role in sperm health. Three additional functions of zinc have been discovered apart from its important antioxidant one:

1. The genetic material (DNA chromatin) in the sperm nucleus is tightly wound with special proteins to form an insoluble, stable complex. This condensed structure is important for successful fertilization. Zinc is important for this structure and protects it from breaking down.
2. The high concentration of zinc in semen damps down sperm activity, keeping them in a relatively quiescent state. This lowers their consumption of oxygen and conserves sperm energy. Once within the female reproductive tract, which contains very

little zinc, zinc concentrations are rapidly diluted. This causes a sudden increase in sperm activity, speeding them up and acting like a mineral turbo charge.

3. During fertilization, a sperm exposes enzymes in a sac at the sperm head to drill a hole in the outer egg shell through which the sperm can pass. This is known as the acrosome reaction. In many cases of subfertility it seems that large numbers of sperm discharge their enzymes spontaneously before or just after ejaculation. By the time they reach the egg they are no longer capable of penetrating it. This early discharge of the acrosome reaction is linked with a zinc deficiency.

    High concentrations of zinc in semen helps to damp down the acrosome reaction in a reversible way. Once zinc concentrations become diluted within the female tract, the acrosome reaction can again occur.

Another recent finding is that zinc deficiency changes the sequence in which seminal secretions are ejaculated. The secretions from the seminal vesicle, which are usually ejaculated last, are released along with the sperm instead.

There are several theories why this happens. Lack of zinc may cause swelling of the prostate gland, which will slow sperm travelling up from the testes. This swelling will also slow the release of prostatic secretions, which are usually the first fluids to be ejaculated.

It is possible that this alteration in the ejaculatory sequence is a survival response to low concentrations of sperm zinc. By mixing the sperm and the relatively zinc-rich seminal vesicle secretions as early as possible, the protective effects of zinc (stabilization of sperm DNA; delaying of acrosome reaction; conservation of energy) are maximized.

Most men do not obtain enough dietary zinc. Those that are highly sexually active may be losing more zinc per day in their semen (5 mg per ejaculation) than they can keep up with in their diet. Men ideally need a minimum of 15 mg zinc from their diet per day *(see pages 354–5)*.

ALCOHOL AND SPERM

As much as 40 per cent of male subfertility has been blamed on moderate alcohol intake. Alcohol damps down testosterone secretion and also hastens its conversion to oestrogen in the liver. This can lead to lowered sperm counts and a decreased sex drive.

Research shows that refraining from alcohol brings sperm counts up to normal within three months in 50 per cent of men with subfertility. Sperm motility also improves.

In one study, 26 men out of 67 (39 per cent) attending a hospital infertility clinic had a low sperm count. All were extensively investigated and no cause for their subfertility was found. These 26 men were advised to stop drinking alcohol and the sperm counts of 13 of them rose to normal within three months. The number of motile sperm increased significantly and the numbers of abnormal forms also dropped. As a result, at least 10 men (78 per cent of those whose sperm counts responded) successfully fathered a child.

EXERCISE AND SPERM

It is well known that excessive exercise can affect the fertility of female athletes by stopping the normal menstrual cycle (a condition known as 'runners' amenorrhoea'). New research shows that overtraining can damp down fertility in males, too.

Fit males who routinely took part in endurance training (e.g. running, swimming, cycling) for more than four days per week were asked to double their average weekly mileage (i.e. to overtrain) for a two-week period.

Their semen and blood hormone levels were analysed for six months before the period of overtraining, again immediately afterwards, and three months later.

Immediately after overtraining, their sperm counts fell by as much as 43 per cent. After three months, sperm counts had dropped to 52 per cent lower than before they overtrained. The number of immature and non-viable sperm increased. All semen samples stayed within the accepted fertile range, however, and this would not be expected to interfere with fertility except where sperm counts were already low.

The blood levels of testosterone hormone also fell significantly by over a third (36 per cent) immediately after overtraining but returned to normal within three months. In contrast, blood levels of the steroid hormone, cortisol, increased by almost 50 per cent.

Cortisol is a steroid secreted in times of stress. It encourages breakdown of muscle and is linked with the muscle wasting that can occur with prolonged overtraining. Cortisol also damps down the secretion of testosterone by Leydig cells in the testis, and is the probable cause of this observed decrease in sperm count. This would also fit in with anecdotal findings that stressed people are less fertile. It is important to realize, however, that the overtraining only occurred for a two-week period in this particular study. The effects of long-term overtraining on male fertility are likely to be more profound.

ENVIRONMENTAL OESTROGENS AND SPERM

Recent research has linked exposure to increased levels of the female hormone, oestrogen, with the observed falling sperm counts.

This is based on the effects of a synthetic oestrogen (diethylstilboestrol) prescribed to millions of pregnant women between 1945 and 1971 to prevent a threatened miscarriage. The male offspring of these pregnancies, who were exposed to diethylstilboestrol in the womb, had an increased risk of undescended testicles, abnormal penis development and future testicular cancers. As adults, they also produced low semen volumes and low sperm counts.

Over the last 30–50 years, these same birth defects have become more common in men who have not knowingly been exposed to synthetic oestrogens in the womb. At the same time, semen volume and sperm counts in adult males have fallen dramatically (*see page 78*). Scientists suggest that men are exposed to weak environmental oestrogens from many sources. These include:

- Foods:
  - plant and fungal hormones (phytoestrogens) such as soya, rye extracts
  - use of anabolic oestrogens in livestock. This was banned in Europe in 1981, but was an important source of exposure in the 1950s–1970s.
  - increased intake of dairy products. Cows continue to lactate while pregnant, so their milk contains high amounts of oestrogen.
- Low-fibre diets, which encourage greater absorption of dietary oestrogens from the stomach and intestines.
- Body fat – which can convert other steroid hormones into oestrogen. Forty-five per cent of British males are now overweight; 8 per cent are obese.
- Pollutants such as PCBs, dioxins, and dichloro-diphenyl trichloroethane. Exhaust gases from petrol engines.
- Traces of drugs (e.g. contraceptive pills; hormone replacement therapy) in drinking water.

These weak environmental oestrogens may have an effect on the developing male foetus and on the rapidly maturing testes at puberty. They are thought to inhibit the division of Sertoli cells in the testes and to inhibit the development of the testicular Leydig cells (*see page 44*).

Sertoli cells are essential for sperm maturation, but each one can only support a certain number of sperm. If there are less Sertoli cells, a lower sperm count is inevitable. Leydig cells manufacture testosterone, and less cells would mean less circulating levels of androgens. This would increase the risk of undescended testes and of future low sperm counts. The environmental oestrogen theory needs further investigation, but observation of animals in the wild seems to back it up. Recent research also suggests that men who drink more milk than usual – and are therefore exposed to higher quantities of cow's oestrogen – are at increased risk of developing testicular cancer (*see page 37*).

DIABETES AND SPERM

Until recently, it was thought that men with diabetes were less fertile than men who did not have diabetes. Recent studies suggest that the opposite may be true – sperm from men with diabetes may be more efficient. They seem to swim in straighter lines and to reach the egg more quickly. The significance of this is not yet fully understood.

CHLAMYDIA AND SPERM

Chlamydia is one of the most common sexually transmissible diseases in the Western world *(see page 163)*. It causes Pelvic Inflammatory Disease (PID) in women and subfertility because it 'furs up' the Fallopian tubes. Research suggests Chlamydia infection can lower fertility in males, too, resulting in a lower sperm count, lower sperm motility and a higher percentage of abnormal sperm than is true of men who are free from infection. These findings are reversible with antibiotics.

HIV AND SPERM

Men who are HIV positive now have a better chance of fathering healthy children without increasing the risk of infecting an HIV-negative partner.

A technique has been perfected to wash semen and separate the sperm from the infective fluids. Motile sperm are then isolated and used for artificial insemination. The technique is estimated to have only a 4 per cent risk of inseminating the mother with infected sperm.

5

INFERTILTIY

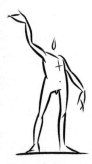

The human male has one of the poorest sperm production rates of any animal on earth. Whereas most animals produce 20–25 million sperm per gram of testicle per day, human males only produce 4 million. The gorilla is even worse, and has a penis and scrotum that are so small they are hardly visible. This may be an evolutionary response to the fact that humans and gorillas are monogamous creatures and there is little male competition to inseminate each female. This cuts out the normal evolutionary processes of survival of the fittest, where the offspring of males with greater sperm production are more likely to be selected out.

For a male to be fertile, he must make normal amounts of motile sperm, transport these through the epididymis and vas deferens and be capable of erection and ejaculation during which sperm are deposited in the vagina of a fertile female. The sperm must then be capable of swimming through the cervical mucus and up into the female's Fallopian tubes to meet a newly ovulated egg. These sperm must be able to identify the egg, stick to its outer coating, expose enzymes that can dissolve through the outer egg shell (acrosome reaction) and thrust forwards through the shell to fertilize the egg. Once fusion has occurred, sperm DNA must be sufficiently normal to allow the embryo to develop.

Male infertility can therefore result from abnormal spermatogenesis, sperm motility, erection, ejaculation or failure of sperm–egg interactions. These processes are so complex it is surprising they do not go wrong more often.

Infertility is defined as the inability to conceive a child after one year of regular, unprotected intercourse.

Infertility affects one in every six couples at some time. For at least 30 per cent of couples seeking treatment, male infertility is the problem; it is a contributory factor in another 20 per cent of cases. Altogether there are around 1 million subfertile males in the UK.

In one study, in which 472 infertile couples were investigated, the cause was identified as:

- a low sperm count in 12 per cent of cases
- total absence of sperm in 6 per cent
- male antibodies to sperm in 8 per cent
- lack of adequate sexual intercourse in a further 6 per cent.

Normal spermatogenesis requires follicle stimulating hormone (FSH), Luteinising hormone (LH) and testosterone hormone. FSH and LH are secreted by the pituitary gland in the brain when a trigger, Gonadotrophin Releasing Hormone (GnRH), is released by another part of the brain, the hypothalamus.

The amounts of FSH and LH secreted are controlled by a clever feedback mechanism involving testosterone. The testosterone feeds back to the pituitary and hypothalamus to reduce the amounts of GnRH and LH that are produced. Another hormone, inhibin, is made by Sertoli cells and also feeds back to control the amount of GnRH and FSH released.

This system of interlinked hormones is complex, and a hormonal imbalance – such as too much inhibin, pituitary failure, or an abnormality of hormone receptors in any of the organs involved – can all result in a failure of spermatogenesis – either producing a low sperm count (oligospermia) or absent sperm (azoospermia).

Other causes of male infertility (or subfertility) include:

- excessive heat or electrostatic electricity around the testicles
- lifestyle problems such as excessive alcohol, smoking and stress
- previous epididymo-orchitis
- previous bilateral mumps orchitis
- untreated low-grade infection (e.g. Chlamydia) with inflammatory cells in the semen
- previous testicular problems (e.g. torsion) or undescended testicle(s)
- congenital malformations, such as lack of ejaculatory ducts, absence of the vas deferens
- blocked epididymes or vas deferens due to scarring, such as after infection with gonorrhoea or Chlamydia
- immobilizing sperm antibodies
- retrograde ejaculation *(see page 108)*
- genetic abnormalities
- impotence
- anti-cancer chemotherapy
- serious illness such as liver or kidney failure

Over the last 50 years, sperm counts have fallen from an average of 113 million sperm per ml to between 66 and 76 million per ml. Semen volume has dropped from an average of 3.4 ml to 2.75 ml, and sperm motility has decreased. Over the last 15 years, the number of men with low sperm counts has tripled, while those with reduced sperm motility doubled from 21 per cent to 43 per cent. Researchers have also found that the number of abnormal sperm (e.g. two heads, two tails, sperm clumped together) has multiplied by a factor of 12. It is now fairly normal to find up to 40 per cent abnormal sperm in a semen analysis.

As a general rule, 50 per cent of men with sperm counts 20–40 million per ml are subfertile, while men with a sperm count lower than 20 million per ml are usually considered sterile. This is not strictly true, however – lower levels of motile sperm are more accurately associated with an increase in the time it takes to achieve fertilization.

Motile sperm count (millions/ml)	Average no. female cycles to conception
<5	11
5–20	9
20–60	8
>60	6

There is a documented case in which a male with a sperm count as low as five thousand motile sperm per ml of semen has successfully fathered a child by natural means. DNA analysis makes him 99.99 per cent certain to be the biological father.

Studies suggest that a man with between 5 and 10 million motile sperm per ml has a 30 per cent chance of eventually fathering a child. When the motile sperm count rises above 100 million per ml, the chance of eventual success increases to 70 per cent.

Relationship of motile sperm count to pregnancy rate among treated infertile couples

Motile sperm count (millions per ml)	Pregnancy rate
<5	33%
5.1–10	28%
10.1–20	53%
20.1–40	57%
40.1–60	60%
60.1–100	63%
>100	70%

Abstaining from ejaculation for 7 to 10 days before the female's peak fertile phase (between 12 and 19 days before her next period is due to start) can improve the chances of conception further. Research shows this increases sperm count while having no significant effect on sperm motility or viability.

A recent study found abnormally high levels of free radicals in semen samples of over half the subfertile males investigated. It was thought these were the by-products of long-term, unrecognized (subclinical) infection that had not produced any symptoms. A commonly responsible organism is Ureoplasma, which was only recently identified in the male tract due to the difficulty in culturing it. It is hoped that treating men affected with this infection with antibiotics and vitamin E (to scavenge the free radicals) will improve their chances of fathering a child.

TIPS TO IMPROVE SPERM COUNT

The following advice will help to optimize male sperm counts. A few simple lifestyle changes are often all that is needed to tip the balance between subfertility and fertility – especially where motile sperm counts are borderline.

- Avoid hot baths and saunas (see page 65).
- Wear loose, cotton boxer shorts (see page 66).
- Regularly splash the testicles with cold water.
- Reduce alcohol intake – preferably to zero. Forty per cent of male subfertility is linked with drinking four units of alcohol per day (see page 74).
- Reduce caffeine intake to no more than three drinks of coffee/tea/cola per day.
- Stop smoking to reduce the amount of free radicals generated (see page 68).
- Lose any excess weight, which tends to cause testosterone/oestrogen imbalances.
- Reduce stress levels by learning relaxation techniques

Obtain adequate amounts of antioxidants in your diet. These mop up free radicals, which account for up to 40 per cent of sperm damage. Ideally, you need:

- at least 250 mg vitamin C per day. Smokers need 500–1000 mg vitamin C per day
- at least 50–100 mg vitamin E per day
- 15 mg betacarotene per day
- 10 mg zinc per day

– this effectively means taking supplements.

THE TREATMENT OF MALE INFERTILITY

Until recently, the only treatment available to help couples where the male had a subfertile motile sperm count was artificial insemination with donor sperm. Their future now looks brighter.

Various investigations may be performed, including analysis of sperm clumping, forward motility, dye tests to establish patency of the vas deferens and epididymes, and testicular biopsy to establish whether spermatogenesis is proceeding normally or not.

There is some evidence that if a male makes antisperm antibodies, these can be damped down with steroid hormones (e.g. prednisolone) which suppresses the immune system, but this has potential side-effects and is not widely practised.

Using male hormones to improve sperm count does not seem to work unless a definite hormone problem was originally identified. Fertility pills equivalent to those given to women (e.g. clomiphene) have also failed to improve fertility.

New techniques that enable a blocked epididymis to be by-passed involve cutting the vas deferens on the affected side, and joining it directly to a sperm collecting tubule within the head of the epididymis with five to six micro-stitches. The technique is known as vasoepididymostomy and successfully leads to pregnancy in 72 per cent of cases. Fertility seems to depend on the motility (i.e. maturity) of sperm coming through rather than their numbers.

Another step forward in treating male infertility was the understanding that some men make sperm that are incapable of exposing the enzymes present in their acrosome sac. These enzymes are essential for the sperm to penetrate an egg. Absence of the acrosome reaction can be overcome by treating the sperm with the antioxidant drug pentoxifylline before artificial insemination. This drug, a caffeine derivative, also acts as a sort of turbo-charge for sluggish sperm and, although its effect is short-lived, it is often enough to allow successful *in vitro* fertilization.

Inadequate zinc levels also trigger the acrosome reaction too

83

early, so sufficient amounts of zinc in the diet are important *(see pages 354–5)*.

Several other recent developments using test-tube fertility techniques have been perfected. Where sperm counts are very low or have poor survival times, sperm can be concentrated by freezing multiple samples, separating out the motile from the im- mobile sperm, and using chemical treatments to increase their fertilizing capacity. One technique involves spinning semen at G forces of 2,000 revolutions per minute and then sieving out the strongest and fastest-swimming ones. This is especially useful for men who have had a reversal of vasectomy with subsequent low sperm counts due to a vas deferens stricture.

The average pregnancy rate achieved with *in vitro* fertilization and embryo transfer techniques is a respectable 17 per cent per treatment cycle. Success rates vary from hospital to hospital, however.

Another technique is intrauterine insemination, in which prepared sperm are injected directly into the uterus. This seems to more than double the chance of fathering a child for those men whose subfertility is caused by a low sperm count.

Where sperm counts are very low, or where sperm seem incapable of piercing an egg (e.g. failure of the acrosome reaction), new fertilization skills allow an egg shell to be thinned (partial zona dissection) or to have a hole drilled through (zona drilling), either by laser or with enzymes pumped through tiny micro-pipettes. Alternatively, sperm can be injected directly under the egg shell using a needle seven times thinner than a human hair. This technique, known as SUZI (subzonal insemination), effectively gets the job done in one fell swoop.

Fertilization rate after SUZI

Motile sperm count (millions)	Eggs fertilized
<1	8%
1–20	20%
>20	30%

A refinement of SUZI allows the sperm to be injected directly into the egg 'white', or cytoplasm. This is known as DISCO (direct injection of sperm into the cytoplasm of the oocyte) or ICSI (intracytoplasmic sperm injection). These techniques are especially useful for non-motile sperm and for sperm with round heads that lack the sac of enzymes (acrosome) necessary for piercing the egg's shell.

One study suggests that DISCO/ICSI fertilization is successful in over 60 per cent of cases, which is higher than the rate of success for SUZI (up to 30 per cent). Pre-embryos then need to be transferred to the mother's womb and achieve implantation for the procedure to result in pregnancy. Problems with implantation can still occur, so the overall success of both SUZI and DISCO is actually 5 per cent, but these figures are improving all the time as new skills are perfected.

Sperm Retrieval

If a physical blockage prevents sperm from being ejaculated (e.g. vasectomy), or if erectile failure is the problem, sperm can be aspirated directly from the epididymis (the convoluted tube between the testis and the vas deferens) using a fine needle. The sperm are then processed by spinning, washing and filtering to concentrate and isolate healthy specimens. These can then be used for artificial insemination within the test-tube, or for any of the techniques described above. This technique has allowed males with severe spinal injury (paralysis and impotence) to father children successfully.

Electrical stimulation can be used to trigger orgasm if the problem is erectile failure or an inability to ejaculate and, in the case of retrograde ejaculation (where sperm are shot backwards into the bladder at orgasm rather than out through the tip of the penis); sperm can be salvaged from the bladder immediately after ejaculation.

DRUGS AND MALE SUBFERTILITY

Drugs which can affect spermatogenesis and lower sperm counts in some men include:

- anticancer treatments (particularly mustargen, cyclophosphamide, chlorambucil), which depress sperm production and lower the numbers of dividing cells
- sulfasalazine, used to treat ulcerative colitis – this reduces sperm motility and density
- ketoconazole, an anti-fungal agent, which may interfere with testosterone action when taken by mouth
- cimetidine, an anti-ulcer drug, which can interfere with testosterone action
- spironolactone, a diuretic, which can interfere with testosterone action
- anabolic steroids *(see page 254)* and corticosteroids, which can significantly lower sperm counts – negative effects may be reversible if the man stops taking them, but after chronic use the damage is often permanent
- antimalarial drugs, which may suppress spermatogenesis
- antihypertensive drugs (beta-blockers, thiazide diuretics), which can cause impotence and low sperm counts
- tricyclic antidepressant drugs and some sedatives, which can cause impotence
- illicit drugs – e.g. opiates and marijuana – can depress spermatogenesis and interfere with the action of GnRH and testosterone.

If you suffer from infertility and are taking any of the above drugs, consult your doctor for advice on stopping or switching them.

If you are due to have anti-cancer chemotherapy, but have not begun or finished having a family, it is worth having sperm samples frozen in a sperm bank before treatment as insurance for the future.

6

THE PROSTATE GLAND

The prostate gland is a time-bomb ticking away deep in the plumbing of every male. The World Health Organization (WHO) estimates that 80 per cent of men will eventually need treatment for prostate problems. One in three will need an operation.

Despite these appalling statistics, few men know where their prostate gland is, what it does, or the symptoms that occur when it starts to go wrong. More importantly, few men realize that a prostate-friendly diet can reduce their risk of developing the three major prostate diseases: benign prostatic hyperplasia, prostatitis, and prostate cancer.

THE HEALTHY PROSTATE GLAND

A healthy prostate gland weighs around 20 g and is the size and shape of a large chestnut. It is made up of millions of tiny glands that secrete a thin, milky, acidic fluid. The prostate also contains muscle and fibre cells which help the gland to contract.

The prostate is hidden away between the bladder and the

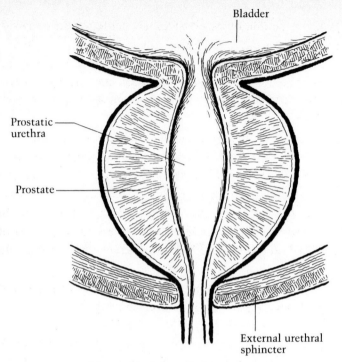

Bladder

Prostatic
urethra

Prostate

External urethral
sphincter

Figure 13: A healthy prostate gland

penis, wrapped around the urethra – the tube through which
urine flows from the bladder. This is a major design flaw: with
increasing age the prostate naturally starts to enlarge. This
squeezes the urethra and interferes with urinary flow.

WHAT DOES THE
PROSTATE GLAND DO?

The function of the prostate gland is not fully understood.
What is known is that the prostate:

- secretes fluids that make up 30–40 per cent of semen volume.
- secretes nutrients such as zinc, amino acids, citric acid, vitamins
  and sugars that are thought to keep sperm healthy, but are not
  essential for reproduction. Sperm which have not come into
  contact with prostate fluid can still fertilize an egg.

- helps to direct semen outwards during ejaculation so sperm don't reflux up into the bladder.
- contains substances that give semen its characteristic smell.
- secretes enzymes such as acid phosphatase and prostatic specific antigen (PSA) which help to increase semen fluidity so sperm can swim away.
- secretes hormone-like chemicals (prostaglandins) which have effects on the female genital tract, such as making the cervix 'pout' slightly so sperm can swim through more easily, and perhaps causing the female tract to contract. In theory this may help 'suck' sperm higher up towards the egg, and may also make the female orgasm more intense. As prostate secretions are the first fluids released during ejaculation, these effects may be important.

Three main things tend to go wrong with the prostate gland; each occurs at a different stage in a man's life:

1. Prostatitis, in which the gland becomes infected or inflamed. This is most common between the ages of 25 and 45.
2. Benign prostatic hyperplasia (BPH), in which the gland slowly enlarges. This commonly causes symptoms after the age of 45.
3. Prostate cancer, which tends to occur over the age of 55 – though it can occur much earlier.

PROSTATITIS

When looked at under a microscope, the prostate gland contains more canals and blind passageways than Venice. These can become infected, inflamed or clogged – either with thickened secretions or tiny, gravel-like stones – to produce prostatitis. It is estimated that one in three men will suffer from prostatitis at some stage between the ages of 20 and 50 years.

There are four main types of prostatitis:

1. acute (recent onset) bacterial infection
2. chronic infection, of one of two kinds:
   a. (long-term, grumbling) bacterial infection

b. (long-term) non-bacterial inflammation
3.   prostatodynia – symptoms of prostate pain without obvious signs of inflammation or infection.

Acute Bacterial Prostatitis

This is usually caused by bacteria from the intestines which find their way into the urinary system either through the urethra or by travelling in the bloodstream or lymphatic fluids.

Sometimes, organisms causing sexually transmissible diseases (e.g. gonorrhoea, Chlamydia) are involved. Occasionally, the fungus that causes thrush (Candida) is responsible too.

Symptoms strike suddenly and can include:

- feeling unwell
- chills or fever
- low back pain
- aching round the thighs and genitals
- deep pain between the scrotum and anus
- pain and difficulty on passing water
- frequency of passing water
- pain on ejaculation

the prostate gland will also usually be hot, swollen and tender when the doctor examines it (by gently inserting a finger in the back passage).

Sometimes, infection persists in the nooks and crannies of the prostate gland, despite treatment. When this happens, chronic prostatitis results.

Chronic Prostatitis

Chronic prostatitis is common in developed countries. Post-mortem studies show that one in five men under the age of 40 years and as many as three in five older males demonstrate evidence of having had the condition. This suggests that chronic (ongoing) inflammation of the prostate gland is often present without causing symptoms.

Studies show that there are two main types of chronic prostatitis, those due to a microbial infection and those in which inflammation is present without any signs of infection.

Chronic Bacterial Prostatitis

Micro-organisms can enter the prostate gland to set up a localized infection with pus and even micro-abscesses. Swelling rapidly occurs, which traps the bacteria in the gland as the usual drainage channels become blocked off.

In some cases, bacteria become coated in prostatic secretions that harden to form tiny crystals or stones. This protects them from attack by the body's immune system and antibiotics and accounts for the repeated flare-ups that are common in chronic bacterial prostatitis.

Symptoms vary, but may include:

- pain and discomfort in the prostate, scrotum, testes, rectum or tip of the penis
- aching in the lower back, lower abdomen or inner thighs
- watery discharge from the penis
- urinary problems such as urgency, getting up at night to pass water, pain on passing water
- pain on ejaculation
- premature ejaculation
- blood in the semen
- infection and swelling of the testes.

Unfortunately, this condition can be difficult to eradicate. Some men suffer recurrent symptoms throughout their life.

Chronic Non-bacterial Prostatitis

This can occur at any time after puberty but is commonest between the ages of 30 and 50. It is an inflammatory condition in which prostate secretions contain white pus cells but no bacteria.

One of the most popular theories is that non-bacterial pro-statitis is due to abnormal emptying of the bladder. This forces urine into the prostate channels and ducts, to cause chemical irritation and inflammation. This is sometimes triggered, or made worse, if a man jogs or plays active sports on a full bladder.

Another theory is that some men produce prostate secretions that are thicker, and perhaps more acid than normal. They cannot drain away through the narrow ducts quite so easily and build up to produce swelling and irritation.

The most common **symptoms** of chronic non-bacterial pro-statitis are:

- pain/ache in the testicles, penis or rectum
- low backache, especially after intercourse
- burning on passing water
- urinary frequency
- discharge from the urethra, especially after sex.

Prostatodynia

Prostatodynia is characterized by pain and symptoms of prostate problems, but with no evidence of inflammation or infection in the gland. Prostate secretions look normal and do not contain pus cells.

Prostatodynia is surprisingly common, accounting for a third of cases where men experience chronic prostatic symptoms.

These **symptoms** often include sexual problems such as:

- pain on erection or ejaculation
- low sex drive
- low semen volume
- impotence.

As a result, some doctors have labelled it a psychosexual problem. It is likely to have a physical cause, however, such as spasm of the pelvic muscles – perhaps brought on by stress and anxiety. Symptoms are often made worse when ejaculation is infrequent, which suggests that the pain may be due to prostatic gland engorgement, perhaps with secretions that are thicker than normal.

Both non-bacterial prostatitis and prostatodynia are sometimes relieved by increased frequency of ejaculation, either through sexual intercourse or masturbation. This drains the gland of excess secretions and temporarily increases blood supply. Both effects help to flush away toxins. In some cases, however, increased frequency of ejaculation just makes the problem worse.

Another possibility is that prostatodynia is due to the irritation or malfunction of the nerves supplying the prostate gland.

How Prostatitis Is Investigated

Prostatitis is frequently difficult to diagnose accurately. It is best investigated by doctors specializing in urology or genito-urinary medicine.

You may well be referred to a special (genito-urinary or VD) clinic, but this doesn't necessarily mean your doctor thinks you have a venereal disease. It's just that genito-urinary clinics have the equipment and expertise to investigate and treat your symptoms sympathetically and in confidence. The tests you are likely to have will include:

- a full genital and rectal examination
- swabs from the end of the penis
- urine cultures and a 'three-glass' test (see below)
- prostatic massage
- a blood test to check for signs of infection (raised white cell count)
- routine screening for sexually transmissible diseases such as Chlamydia.

During examination, the doctor will look for a discharge from the end of the penis and signs of inflammation such as redness or soreness. The testicles may be gently examined for lumps or tenderness.

A rectal examination is usually performed to assess the gland's size and texture, but this is not always helpful. In acute prostatitis the prostate is usually hot, swollen or tender. In chronic prostatitis it may feel boggy and soft, but often seems perfectly normal.

Swabs are taken by gently inserting a sterile cotton bud into the end of the penis. This collects fresh discharge which is then examined under the microscope before being sent for bacterial culture.

A second swab is sent for special analysis to detect signs of Chlamydia infection. Unlike normal bacteria, Chlamydia are too small to be seen under a light microscope and cannot be grown in culture.

Urine tests for Prostatitis

You will be asked to provide a urine sample by passing a small amount of water into one glass jar, and more into a second jar.

These samples are checked for cloudiness, signs of protein or blood, and for threads of cellular material. Threads are fished out for examination under the microscope, as the presence of pus cells or bacteria can help with the diagnosis. The remaining urine is sent for culture to see if any bacteria grow.

Usually, a 'three-glass' test is done. After passing urine into the second jar, you are asked to stop voiding and retain some urine. The doctor then inserts a gloved finger into your rectum and gently massages the prostate gland.

Massaging the gland releases secretions which can be milked down to the tip of the penis and collected. If no fluid appears, you will be asked to pass a small sample of urine into a third glass jar to flush the released prostate fluids through.

ANALYSIS OF THE THREE GLASS TEST

The three-glass test aims to distinguish between infection in different parts of the male urogenital tract. The results are not always clear cut, but in general they may be summarized as follows:

- If bacteria are found in the first glass jar, this suggests infection of the urethra (the tube leading from the bladder to the tip of the penis).
- If bacteria are present in the second sample, this suggests you might have a bladder infection (cystitis).
- If more bacteria are found in the third glass jar than in the first, this suggests prostatitis.
- If pus cells are present, but no significant bacteria are found in any sample, this suggests non-bacterial prostatitis.
- If no bacteria and very few pus cells are found, the diagnosis may be prostatodynia.

Treatment of Prostatitis

Acute Prostatitis

Once the diagnosis is made, a prolonged course of antibiotic tablets are prescribed, usually for at least four weeks. Symptoms should start to improve within a few days.

Occasionally, infection causes the gland to swell enough to squeeze the urethra shut. This causes urinary outflow obstruction, and admission to hospital is required. A catheter is inserted into the bladder under local anaesthetic to ease the urinary flow.

Chronic Prostatitis

Chronic infection can be difficult to treat, as inflammation and swelling traps infection inside the gland. Once the diagnosis is made, antibiotics are prescribed for at least six weeks. Sometimes, they are needed for three months or more.

Anti-inflammatory painkillers such as ibuprofen also help to damp down swelling, inflammation and pain.

Chronic non-bacterial prostatitis can be treated with a natural food supplement derived from rye pollen extracts. This has been shown to reduce inflammation, irritation and swelling. First signs of improvement usually show within three months, and there is a progressive improvement over a six-month period.

Prostatodynia

This can be difficult to treat. Painkillers are not usually very helpful and some patients end up on tranquillizers to reduce muscular spasm in the gland. These are not a good idea for long-term use as they can become addictive.

Recent studies suggest that prostate pain is relieved by microwave hyperthermia. The prostate gland is warmed from 37 to 42.5°C (98.6 to 108.5°F) by a special instrument inserted into the back passage. This increases the blood supply and speeds up the body's natural healing reactions. An hour's treatment is given for six weeks.

Similar relief is sometimes obtained by sitting in a hot bath for half an hour.

Other treatments which have been tried for prostatodynia include:

- acupuncture
- laser irradiation
- muscle relaxant drugs (e.g. diazepam)
- anti-spasmodic drugs
- psychotherapy and counselling
- relaxation techniques

Regular exercise and a high-fibre diet to keep the bowels regular are important for men with prostatodynia, especially if they sit at a desk for most of the day. Both sitting and constipation increase prostate congestion.

The nicotine in cigarettes causes spasm of smooth muscle and may exacerbate the symptoms of prostatodynia. Alcohol or caffeine can also trigger attacks of prostate pain, and it might be worth seeing an allergy specialist to identify foods you should avoid.

Prostatitis and Sex

If you suffer from prostatitis it is best to avoid sex while you have symptoms or are taking treatment. If the problem is due to infection, it is theoretically possible to pass this on to cause cystitis or vaginal infection in a female partner. Your doctor will advise on when you can resume normal sexual relations.

BENIGN PROSTATIC ENLARGEMENT

The prostate gland naturally enlarges with increasing age. This process is known as benign prostatic hyperplasia, usually abbreviated to BPH.

As a rough estimate, one in three men over the age of 50 have symptoms of prostatism. It becomes increasingly common with advancing age (so that by 60 years of age, 60 per cent of men have clinical symptoms; by the age of 70, 70 per cent have symptoms, and so on.)

Unfortunately (as mentioned earlier), since the symptoms tend to creep up slowly many men assume they are just a part of growing old and do not seek investigation or treatment.

The term *hyperplasia* refers to an increase in the number of cells present in the prostate gland. As the number of cells increases, the prostate gland enlarges. Since the prostate encircles the tube through which urine passes to the outside world (the urethra), BPH causes varying degrees of urinary outflow obstruction.

In some men, the prostate gland grows large without causing problems with passing water. This is because their urethra is wider than average, or because the gland tends to enlarge outwards rather than inwards on itself.

In other men, the slightest increase in size means the urethra is compressed, and embarrassing urinary symptoms arise. Doctors call these symptoms *prostatism*.

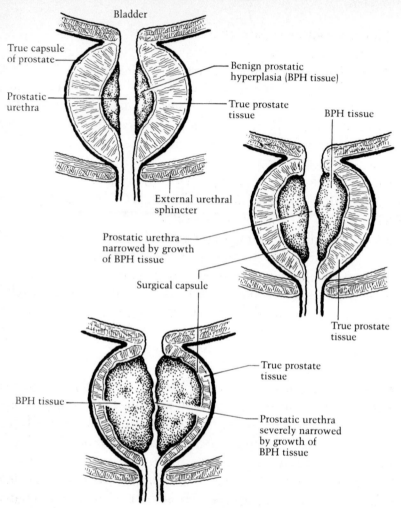

Figure 14: Prostate and urethra, showing central area enlarging as in the case of a) mild BPH, b) moderate BPH, and c) severe BPH

Symptoms of Prostatism

The classic symptoms of prostatism are a combination of urinary outflow obstruction and symptoms due to bladder irritation, as the bladder stretches and thickens as it tries to force urine past the prostatic obstruction. The **symptoms** (• = obstructive symptoms; •• = irritative bladder symptoms) include:

- difficulty starting to pass water (hesitancy)
- a weak stream
- starting and stopping in the middle of passing water
- having to strain to pass water
- dribbling of urine
- incontinence
- urinary retention
- • discomfort when passing water
- • having to rush urgently to the toilet to pass water
- • having to pass water more often
- • having to get up at night to pass water
- • a feeling of not having emptied the bladder fully

NB Blood in the urine or sperm is not usually a symptom of BPH. If you notice either, you must see your doctor as soon as possible as it will need immediate investigation.

What Causes BPH?

Benign prostatic hyperplasia can be blamed on the male sex hormone, testosterone. This is broken down in the prostate gland to another hormone, dihydro-testosterone (DHT). This conversion is controlled by the prostate enzyme 5-alpha-reductase.

Males who lack the 5-alpha-reductase enzyme do not develop normally. Their male genitalia are small and they are usually mistaken for girls until puberty. The penis and scrotum then suddenly enlarge and the voice deepens, which is obviously traumatic for the child, his parents, and all concerned.

Interestingly, these males:

- only develop a tiny prostate gland
- do not go bald
- never suffer from acne.

As it is the breakdown product of testosterone hormone which causes benign prostatic enlargement in later life, prostate problems can be treated by inhibiting the 5-alpha-reductase enzyme which normally triggers this breakdown.

If left untreated, BPH can have serious consequences. Trapped urine can flow back up from the bladder to put pressure on the kidneys. Scarring and damage may eventually result in kidney failure. Although this is uncommon, it illustrates that BPH needs to be taken seriously and not just accepted as an inevitable part of growing old.

International Prostate Symptoms Score

Recently, a working party from the World Health Organization (WHO) drew up a 'prostate symptoms score'. This is a major advance as it provides an objective (rather than subjective) method of gauging the severity of your prostate symptoms.

Look at the chart on the opposite page and work out your own prostate score.

As a general guide, if you score:

- Less than 9: you may not need treatment but will be closely monitored by your doctor to see how your symptoms progress. You may find a prostate-friendly diet or rye pollen extracts helpful.
- 9–17: You have moderate symptoms of BPH. Your doctor may prescribe a drug treatment – provided that your blood levels of prostate specific antigen (PSA – *see page 113*) and digital rectal examination are normal.
- Greater than 17 (or PSA or rectal examination abnormal): you will be referred to a specialist for further investigation and treatment.

Acute Retention of Urine

Eventually, as the prostate continues to enlarge, the urethra may be blocked off altogether. This is often triggered by spasm of the bladder or the pelvic muscles surrounding the urethra. Discomfort and worry about not being able to pass water make the spasm worse. As urine builds up in the bladder, stretch pains become unbearable and admission to

Figure 15: INTERNATIONAL PROSTATE SYMPTOMS SCORE

	Not at all all	Less than one time in five	Less than half the time	About half the time	More than half the time	Almost always
Over the past month how often have you:						
Had a sensation of not completely emptying your bladder after urinating?	0	1	2	3	4	5
Needed to urinate again within two hours of finishing urinating?	0	1	2	3	4	5
Stopped and started again several times when you urinated?	0	1	2	3	4	5
Found it difficult to postpone urination?	0	1	2	3	4	5
Had a weak urinary stream?	0	1	2	3	4	5
Had to push or strain to begin urinating?	0	1	2	3	4	5
Had to get up to urinate from the time you went to bed at night until the time you got up in the morning?	0	1	2	3	4	5

hospital is usually needed.

A tube (catheter) is passed into the bladder, through the penis (under local anaesthetic) to drain trapped urine and bring instant relief. Very rarely the catheter cannot be passed through the urethra due to gross swelling of the prostate gland. If this happens, the urethra can sometimes be gently dilated with special rods. If this fails, a suprapubic catheter can be passed into the bladder through the overlying abdominal wall.

Hopefully, with increased awareness of prostate problems, fewer men will present at this late stage with urinary retention – an extremely embarrassing, unpleasant and painful condition.

BPH and Lifestyle

The symptoms of BPH can have a drastic effect on lifestyle. Common complaints are:

- having to avoid drinking at certain times, such as before an outing or before going to bed
- having to reduce total fluid intake
- having to make sure that you always know where the nearest toilet is
- not participating in social or leisure activities because of fear of embarrassment
- feeling depressed, with low self-esteem.

A recent poll of around one thousand men over the age of 50 found that 27 per cent had to get up at night to pass water. Of these, 13 per cent had put up with the problem for over 10 years. Twenty per cent had difficulty in starting to pass water, and 15 per cent reported frequency. Many men suffered limitation of their social, leisure and sexual activities because of their symptoms.

A MORI poll of 800 men over the age of 50 years showed that:

- Almost half of sexually active males with symptoms of prostatism experience a lowered sex drive, difficulty in sustaining an erection and ejaculatory problems.
- 20 per cent of men with symptoms of BPH had sex at least once per week, compared with 40 per cent of men without symptoms.
- Men with two or more symptoms of prostatism said they would like to have sex more often than their symptoms allowed.

What to Do If You Think You Have BPH

If you suspect you have symptoms of prostatism it is important to consult your doctor straightaway. Don't wait until the symptoms start interfering with your life. Early screening will help to prevent future problems with your kidneys – and will also increase the likelihood that the more serious problem, prostate cancer, is picked up and treated early.

Rectal Examination

Some men admit to not going to their doctor with prostate symptoms because they dread the thought of a rectal examination.

The size, shape, texture and tenderness of the prostate gland can be assessed by the doctor gently inserting a finger into your back passage. This is called a digital rectal examination, usually abbreviated to DRE, and it is nowhere near as unpleasant as many men think. Most patients describe the sensation as similar to slight constipation.

The doctor uses a colourless, odourless, water-based jelly as a lubricant. Only the index finger is inserted – which, if you think about it, is much thinner than the width of the average bowel motion.

CONDITION	DRE FINDINGS
Prostatitis	soft, boggy and tender
BPH	enlarged, smooth, firm
	anatomical groove may be felt
Prostate Cancer	hard nodular, craggy feel to gland
	loss of normal anatomical groove

Investigation of an Enlarged Prostate Gland

Blood Tests

- Full Blood Count to check for anaemia or infection
- Urea and Electrolytes – to check how well your kidneys are working.
- Prostate Specific Antigen (PSA) – which may be raised if there is a hidden prostate tumour *(see page 113)*

- Prostatic acid phosphatase (PAP) – which may be raised in prostate cancer if secondary cancers have spread to the bones

Urine Tests

- Urine 'dip-stick' test – to check for sugar and protein
- Mid-Stream Urine (MSU) – to check for bacterial infection (cystitis), red blood cells, pus cells and casts (minute threads of tissue shed from the kidney)
- Urinary flow rate – to assess how badly your stream is affected. This involves passing urine into a bottle with a special by-pass, or into a funnel with an electronic device attached. The speed you pass urine and the total amount passed are printed out in the form of a graph. This will show how much your urinary outflow is obstructed.

Ultrasound

Ultrasonography passes high-frequency, inaudible sound waves through your body. These bounce back off tissue planes and are analysed by a computer which produces an image on a screen. Ultrasound can check:

- the size of your prostate gland
- the size of your kidneys
- how much residual urine stays in your bladder after voiding
- trans-rectal ultrasonography, in which a lubricated, finger-shaped probe is gently inserted in the back passage, can give a better assessment of the prostate gland and whether enlargement is due to benign hyperplasia or cancer.

Cystoscopy

A narrow telescope (cystoscope) is inserted through the penis into the bladder, under general anaesthetic. This allows assessment of the urethra, the bladder, and the degree of prostate obstruction.

Intravenous Pyelogram (IVP, IVU, excretory urogram)

This test, used only occasionally, involves injecting a radio-opaque form of iodine into a vein, which is then concentrated by the kidneys. X-rays are taken which outline the urinary tract and reveal abnormalities.

Treatment of BPH

Treatment depends on the severity of your symptoms and how much they interfere with your life. The WHO Prostate Symptoms Score *(see Figure 15, page 101)* now allows an objective assessment.

Mild Symptoms

If prostatic enlargement is slight, the treatment approach is one of 'wait and see', so long as the assessment has ruled out malignancy. In some cases symptoms will not get dramatically worse. A prostate-friendly diet and rye pollen extracts may help.

Moderate Symptoms

ANTI-SPASMODIC DRUGS

These drugs (e.g. oxybutinin; flavoxate; propantheline) reduce irritation and spasm of the bladder and help symptoms such as frequency of passing urine, urgency and incontinence. They should not be used if the prostate is greatly enlarged, however, so are of limited value in treating BPH.

ALPHA-BLOCKER DRUGS

These (e.g. prazosin; terazosin; indoramin) damp down activity in the nervous system, which would normally trigger contraction of muscle fibres in the prostate and urethra. By relaxing the muscles, the urethral bore is widened to improve symptoms.

5-ALPHA-REDUCTASE INHIBITORS

These drugs (e.g. finasteride) block the enzyme that converts the male hormone testosterone to dihydro-testosterone – the hormone responsible for BPH *(see page 97)*. This can help an enlarged prostate gland to shrink by over 20 per cent and is particularly beneficial to men with severe symptoms. Treatment needs to be taken continuously as the prostate can start to enlarge within a few weeks of stopping the tablets. Condoms should be used during intercourse while taking these drugs to protect female sexual partners from exposure to the drug, which may be present in the semen.

HORMONES

Hormonal factors influencing prostate symptoms are not fully understood. Treatment with a synthetic progestogen (gestronol) is sometimes given as an injection every five to seven days. It is not commonly used, however, as few men welcome regular injections. Other hormone preparations (e.g. flutamide, cyproterone) have been shown to shrink the prostate gland by 25 per cent but do not significantly improve urinary flow rate or reduce the amount of residual urine remaining in the bladder after voiding. Experts believe it is unlikely that a single hormone treatment will work against BPH.

NATURAL TREATMENTS

Several natural plant products, collectively known as phytotherapy, are used to treat BPH. Like conventional drugs, these have different actions on the prostate gland to improve symptoms. Some shrink or soften the gland to open up the urethra; others relax muscle fibres and reduce spasm of the prostate and bladder.

Europeans have led the field in natural prostate treatments. In Germany, phytotherapy is prescribed for 95 per cent of patients undergoing medical treatment for BPH. In France and Italy, natural plant extracts are used by around 40 per cent of men with symptoms that warrant intervention.

These natural treatments include preparations of:

- South African stargrass – Harzol
- Golden Rod (*Solidago*)

- African prune (*Pygeum africanum*) – Tadenan
- American Dwarf palmetto (*Serenoa repens*) – Permixon
- Rye pollen extracts – Cernilton, ProstaBrit

The two latter plant extracts are interesting as they are thought to inhibit the enzyme 5-alpha- reductase, and reduce inflammation. Sixty-nine per cent of men using rye pollen extracts notice an improvement in symptoms, and their prostate volume shrinks by up to 30 per cent.

SAW PALMETTO: HERBAL TREATMENT FOR AN ENLARGED PROSTATE GLAND

New research confirms that extracts from the fruit of the Saw palmetto (*Sabal serrulata* or *Serenoa repens*) are an effective herbal treatment for symptoms due to benign enlargement of the prostate gland (benign prostatic hyperplasia – BPH). Saw palmetto strengthens the neck of the bladder, shrinks an enlarged prostate gland, and helps to improve urinary flow and bladder voiding. It is thought to work in a number of ways:

- by blocking two prostate enzymes: 5-alpha-reductase and 3-ketosteroid reductase
- by interfering with hormone receptors in the gland so the activity of dihydrotestosterone and oestrogen is reduced
- by relaxing smooth muscle cells in the gland and bladder neck.

These actions help the gland to shrink and relax so urinary flow is improved. Studies show a significant improvement in both day and night time urinary frequency plus a significant increase in urinary flow rate in men taking Saw palmetto extracts for 60 days. A randomized, controlled trial comparing extracts of saw palmetto with a prescription-only drug (finasteride) used to treat BPH showed both treatments achieved a 38 per cent decrease in symptoms over a six-month period. Interestingly, however, sexual function in the men using the natural treatment did not change, although it deteriorated significantly in those taking the prescribed medication. Saw palmetto extracts, therefore, seem to be as effective as the prescribed drug for relieving symptoms of BPH, but without the undesirable side-effects of low sex drive and impotence.

Dose

Fruit extracts: 150 mg – 3 g daily in divided doses.
Products standardized for 85 – 95 per cent fat-soluble sterols: 320 mg daily.

A beneficial effect usually starts within two to six weeks. No significant side-effects have been reported. Saw palmetto (Sabalin) can be obtained by mail order in the UK from Medic Herb (01628 487780).

EVENING PRIMROSE OIL

Evening primrose oil (EPO) is a rich source of an essential fatty acid, gammalinolenic acid (GLA) which can help a wide range of problems including dry, itchy skin, acne, irritable bowel syndrome, rheumatoid arthritis and post-viral fatigue syndrome. It is also helpful for men with benign prostatic hyperplasia (BPH). Like Saw palmetto, it can inhibit an enzyme (5-alpha-reductase) linked with enlargement of the prostate gland, and slow the growth of fibrous tissue. A supplement combining evening primrose oil with Saw palmetto and beta-sitosterol (a plant hormone-like substance) is now also available (Efaprost). For more information, contact the Efamol Information Line (01483 570248).

Severe Symptoms

Traditionally, surgery is the gold standard treatment for moderate to severe benign prostatic hyperplasia. Removal of part or all of the prostate gland has been practised for over a hundred years.

CATHETERIZATION

Catheterization is the insertion of a flexible tube into the bladder to release trapped urine. This can be left in place to provide continual drainage into a bag worn attached to the leg. This option is useful for treating dribbling incontinence but is not acceptable to many men except as a temporary measure. Catheterization is also used as an emergency procedure to release trapped urine in the bladder if the urethra becomes completely blocked.

TRANSURETHRAL PROSTATECTOMY (TURP)

Over 45,000 men in the UK undergo a TURP each year. In the US, over 400,000 are performed every year, at an annual cost of $4 billion.

During a TURP, an instrument (resectoscope) is inserted through the penis while the patient is under a general anaesthetic. A fibre-optic light and lens system allows the surgeon to view the urethra and bulging inner surface of the prostate gland. A high-frequency electric arc is used to trim excess tissue and cauterize bleeding points at the same time. The surgeon pares away the enlarged central portion of the prostate gland from the inside out. A continuous fluid irrigation system flushes the trimmings away and allows some to be collected for examination under a microscope. Histology reveals a hidden tumour in about 5 per cent of cases.

The latest refinement of the TURP is the use of a right-angled laser-fibre. This allows the surgeon to target the prostate tissue for removal more accurately, reducing the risk of complications such as absorption of irrigation fluid, bleeding, incontinence and retrograde ejaculation (see below). Endoscopic laser ablation, as this procedure is known, is currently undergoing trials and may eventually replace the classic TURP.

After a TURP

It usually takes several weeks for symptoms of prostatism to settle down after the operation. Up to 20 per cent of men will have post-operative problems, including intermittent, dribbling incontinence of urine. In about 5 per cent of cases, this problem is continual. Incontinence after the operation is not necessarily irreversible or permanent, however. It generally improves with time and often improves with medication. If necessary, artificial valves may be implanted to relieve the problem.

The prostate gland can still continue enlarging after the

109

operation, so that symptoms eventually recur. Around 15 per cent of men need a second TURP within eight years of the first.

TURP and Sex

It is important to know that at least a third of men undergoing a TURP will suffer retrograde ejaculation after the operation. Some studies suggest the figure is as high as 90 per cent. With retrograde ejaculation sperm are passed backwards into the bladder during orgasm, so very little is ejaculated from the penis. This in itself is not harmful, however, and the sperm will be voided next time you empty your bladder. What it does mean, though, is that you are likely to be subfertile. While it is possible to aspirate sperm from the bladder and use these for artificial insemination techniques, if you think you might want more children in the future it is worth having sperm samples frozen and stored in a sperm bank before the operation. Marie Stopes and The British Pregnancy Advisory Service (see Useful Addresses chapter) offers this facility.

There is no obvious reason why a TURP should affect a man's sex drive or ability to maintain an erection. Never - theless, a few men do seem to experience sexual problems after the operation. Fifty per cent report noticing a change in the intensity of their orgasms, and this may of course make some less interested in sex.

As a general rule, however, you should not fear having erectile problems after a prostate operation. If any do occur, you will be treated as if you haven't had a prostate operation – that is, other causes will be sought.

OPEN PROSTATECTOMY

An open prostatectomy, in which the entire prostate gland is shelled out through an incision over the pubic bone, was the standard prostate operation until TURP was perfected. It is now more widely used in the US than in the UK, where it makes up around only 4 per cent of prostatectomies.

It is still sometimes performed if:

- the prostate is very much enlarged (over 70 g)

- the hip joints are badly affected by arthritis and cannot be placed up in stirrups as required for TURP
- a suspected early tumour might be cured through removal of the entire gland
- large bladder stones also need removal.

The risk of retrograde ejaculation with open prostatectomy is around 80 per cent.

OTHER OPTIONS

Many new procedures have been developed to treat BPH. Not all are widely available and some are still at the clinical trial stage:

TULIP

Trans-urethral, Ultra-sound guided, Laser-Induced Prostatec-tomy. A laser probe is inserted into the urethra as far as the prostate gland. A water-filled balloon is inflated to fix it in place and to help drain blood out of the gland. The bloodless prostate is trimmed and sealed using the laser, which cuts down blood flow even further, causing the gland to shrivel. The procedure causes relatively little bleeding. Only 5 per cent of treated males suffer retrograde ejaculation after this operation.

Stent Implants

A tubular metal mesh implanted in the prostatic urethra is expanded to hold the urethral walls open. Positioning is a minor procedure that takes less than 15 minutes. Two types of stent are available:

1. a fine, tubular wire mesh (Wallstent) that stays in permanently
2. a gold- or silver-plated metal spiral (Fabian urospiral) that is replaced every few years.

Balloon Dilation

A balloon is inserted into the urethra and inflated to dilate the passage through the prostate gland. Initial results seemed promising, but some doubt was recently cast on the effective-ness of this procedure.

Microwave Hyperthermia (Prostatron)

For this technique a microwave coil within a catheter is inserted into the urethra and heated to a temperature of 42°C (107.6°F). A cooling system protects surrounding tissues. The procedure is performed under local anaesthetic and takes between one and two hours. It improves symptoms of BPH by two-thirds and cuts in half the number of times the sufferer has to get up in the night to pass urine.

Transrectal Hyperthermia (Prostathermer)

A probe is introduced into the rectum to heat the prostate gland to a temperature of 42°C (107.6°F) using microwaves. This procedure must be repeated six times to be effective.

Thermex

A radio-frequency device that is still under trials. This only needs to be used once and can treat two patients simultaneously.

TUNA: Trans-Urethral Needle Ablation

Needles are inserted into the prostate gland (under a local anaesthetic) to achieve greater precision and higher temperatures during thermal treatment to shrink the prostate gland.

Sonoblate

A device is inserted via the rectum to focus ultrasound waves on the prostate gland. Temperatures high enough to shrink the gland are produced.

Cryotherapy

Deep Freeze Treatment. A cryoprobe is inserted into the penis as far as the prostate gland. The tip of the instrument is then frozen using liquid nitrogen. This forms a ball of ice that envelops and freezes the prostate gland. After five to 10 minutes the probe is electrically rewarmed and the water content of the gland melts and is flushed away. This produces dramatic shrinkage.

CANCER OF THE PROSTATE GLAND

Cancer of the prostate gland kills three times as many men as cervical cancer kills women – yet there is much less awareness about this common disease.

In the UK, 11,500 new cases are diagnosed every year. In the US it is the commonest diagnosed male malignancy (excluding skin cancers), with 122,000 new cases each year. It is the second most common fatal male tumour and the leading cause of cancer deaths in men over the age of 55.

It is estimated that one in every 11 white American males will develop clinically significant prostate cancer at some stage of their lives. The risk for black males is even higher, with one in every 10 eventually affected.

Autopsy studies show that an astonishing 10–30 per cent of men aged 50–60 years, and 50–70 per cent of men aged 70–80 years, show evidence of prostate cancer when glands are examined under the microscope. Most of these cancers remain silent and are never diagnosed. Their owners die with them, rather than from them.

The incidence of prostate cancer found in autopsies is identical among American, Japanese and Chinese men, but for some reason the cancer is more likely to progress to cause symptoms in Western males. The incidence of recognized disease is 26-fold lower in Chinese men and 10-fold lower among Japanese men. When Japanese men emigrate to the US, their risk of developing clinically significant prostate cancer becomes the same as for American men within two generations. This suggests an environmental factor is involved in converting hidden prostate cancers to clinically significant disease. The most likely culprit is the Western diet.

An Hereditary Disease

Cancer of the prostate gland seems to run in families. If a first-degree relative (father or brother) is affected, a man's risk of developing prostate cancer is almost three times greater than

113

normal. If a second-degree relative (uncle or grandfather) has prostate cancer as well, a man's risk increases to six times that of a male with no affected relatives.

Symptoms of Prostate Cancer

Unfortunately there are usually no symptoms in the early stages of prostate cancer. This is because 90 per cent of tumours arise on the outside of the gland and do not obstruct urinary flow initially. Prostate cancer is slow growing and may take as long as four years to double in size. Sometimes a tumour is picked up early because of coincidental symptoms of benign prostatic hyperplasia (BPH – *see page 97*).

At a later stage of the disease, a man might notice symptoms of obstruction similar to those of benign prostatic hyperplasia. If the disease spreads (metastasis) to other parts of the body – most commonly to bone – symptoms and signs such as the following may develop:

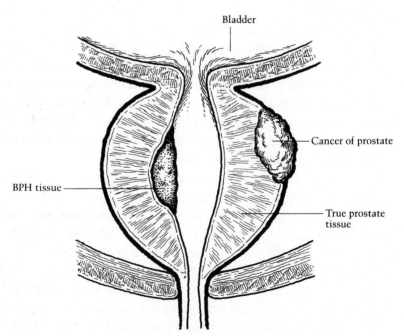

Figure 16: Prostate gland showing BPH plus tumour

- tiredness
- loss of appetite
- weight loss
- bone pain
- anaemia
- blood in the urine or sperm
- swollen glands.

In the UK, only 15 per cent of treatable prostate cancers are picked up in the early stages, compared to 50 per cent in the US where annual screening methods are practised. Screening can take the form of:

- routine blood tests to measure Prostate Specific Antigen (PSA)
- routine digital rectal examinations
- routine Trans-rectal Ultrasound (TRUS) examination of the prostate gland – see below.

Diagnosis

In 90 per cent of cases, a cancer arises in the outer part of the prostate gland where it is felt as a small, hard lump or irregularity during a digital rectal examination. If your doctor does find a lump, try not to worry. In half of all cases referred for urgent investigation, no cancer is found – the lump is due to a stone or other benign enlargement. Even if cancer is present, if caught early enough it is often curable.

If cancer is suspected, several blood tests may be performed to check for anaemia and to assess kidney function. Measuring the level of a blood enzyme known as Prostatic Acid Phosphatase (PAP) is useful to indicate whether a prostate tumour has spread to form bone secondary cancers.

Prostate Specific Antigen (PSA) is a protein made only by prostate cells. If the level of PSA in the blood is above 10 ng/ml there is a 60 per cent chance that cancer of the prostate is present. If the level is moderately raised (between 4 and 10 ng/ml) there is a 20 per cent chance of prostate cancer. This is because other conditions such as benign enlargement or even a digital rectal examination sometimes elevate the level. The only way to distinguish between them is via a biopsy.

If PSA is normal (less than 4 ng/ml) there is only a 2.5 per cent chance that a man has prostate cancer.

Other Tests

Trans-rectal Ultrasound (TRUS)

This involves inserting a lubricated finger-shaped probe into the back passage. Sound waves are passed through the prostate gland and bounce back off tissue planes to form a computer-interpreted image. Tumours often show up as abnormal echoes. Unfortunately, this is not helpful if the cancer has the same echoing qualities as the surrounding normal tissues. A proportion of tumours are therefore missed.

Biopsy

Taking a biopsy is the best way to determine whether a prostate nodule is benign or malignant. A fine needle is used to remove a small sample of tissue from the tumour (under local anaesthetic). If the needle is inserted through the back passage, you may be given antibiotics to prevent infection. Sometimes the needle is guided into the lump using ultrasound. Tissue obtained during the biopsy is then examined under a microscope to look for cancerous cells.

Body Scans

(CAT or MRI) are useful to see how far a tumour has infiltrated surrounding tissues and to check if it has spread into pelvic lymph nodes.

Isotope Bone Scan

As advanced prostate tumours commonly spread to bone, an isotope bone scan is performed once prostate cancer is diagnosed. Bone secondary cancers (secondaries) can also be seen on plain X-rays. Occasionally, the disease is only suspected at a late stage after bone pain or fracture has occurred.

Treatment

Treatment varies from patient to patient and from specialist to specialist. It depends on how advanced the cancer is and whether or not it has spread beyond the prostate gland. Once the disease has spread beyond the gland, treatment is aimed at controlling the condition rather than curing it.

Medical Treatment

Prostate cancers often shrink if their hormone environment is changed. Synthetic hormones that block testosterone (e.g. cyproterone acetate, flutamide) or that mimic a female environment (e.g. oestrogen derivatives) are used to damp down the disease. Unfortunately, female hormones can lead to male breast enlargement, and also reduce the male sex drive.

The male hormone testosterone is only made by the testicles if it receives a hormone signal from the brain. The latest hormone treatments (LHRH agonists e.g. buserelin, goserelin, leuprorelin) act directly on the brain – often via a nasal spray – to prevent this signal being given. This results in a so-called 'chemical castration' as the testicles stop producing testosterone. Unfortunately, side-effects of hot flushes, low sex drive and impotence are inevitable. A third of patients suffer a flare-up of disease symptoms in the first few weeks of treatment as testosterone levels initially go high before petering out.

Radiotherapy may be used to shrink the prostate gland, or to relieve the pain of bone secondaries. This takes the form of external beam irradiation or of radioactive iodine seeds placed in the gland itself. Radioactive bone-seeking substances (e.g. strontium) are beneficial in men with widespread bone secondaries. Unfortunately, chemotherapy with anti-cancer drugs is generally unhelpful.

117

Surgical Treatment

Removal of the testicles (orchidectomy) is occasionally performed in a drastic attempt to lower testosterone levels. If surgical castration is thought necessary, egg-shaped implants may be inserted in the scrotum which look and feel like the real thing.

Side-effects of the operation include hot flushes (similar to those of menopausal women), impotence, loss of libido and adverse psychological effects. Most men would prefer a chemical (hormonal) castration to a surgical one.

If the prostate tumour is small and localized, the whole gland is sometimes removed (radical prostatectomy) in the hope of curing the disease. This operation is done more frequently in the US than in the UK. A recent modification of the operation spares nerve bundles lying close to the prostate gland. This reduces the risk of sexual dysfunction and incontinence.

A new surgical procedure using a YAG laser to remove a malignant prostate gland shows promising early results.

Other treatments currently being investigated include cryotherapy (freezing the gland) and Microwave Hyperthermia (see pages 173 and 112).

The Future

Exciting new research has discovered substances called *bolstered tumour-fighting growth factors* within the prostate gland. These are natural substances produced by the prostate cells as part of the body's tumour-defence mechanism. Although treatment with these factors is a long way off, they offer an exciting possibility for manipulating prostate cancer successfully.

Another possible route to curing prostate cancer is by switching off cancer genes through gene therapy, although it will probably be at least 10 years before this treatment is available.

DIET AND PROSTATE DISEASE

The idea of eating for a healthy heart is now medically accepted – but the concept of eating for a healthy prostate is revolutionary.

Recent studies suggest that this is not only possible – but an important factor in the observed low incidence of prostate disease in certain parts of the world.

Men in China and Japan are less likely to develop prostate cancer, benign prostatic enlargement and prostatitis than Western males. This does not seem to be an inherited trait, as autopsy studies show they have just as high an incidence of hidden prostate cancer as American men. Something in the Eastern lifestyle seems to damp down prostate conditions so they do not progress into clinically significant disease.

If Eastern males move to the West, their prostate protection is lost. There is also evidence that Japanese males who do not emigrate, but who adopt a more Western diet, lose their traditional protection against prostatic disease.

One theory gaining in popularity is that the Eastern diet protects against prostate disease, while a Western-style diet is more likely to trigger prostate problems.

Dietary Plant Oestrogens

The traditional Japanese diet is low in fat, especially saturated fat, and consists of rice, soy products (e.g. soybeans, soymeal, tofu) and fish together with legumes, grains and cruciferous plants. The latter include exotic members of the cabbage and turnip families (e.g. kohlrabi; Chinese leaves). These are all rich in weak plant hormones (isoflavonoids, phytoestrogens) that are released during digestion – probably through bacterial fermentation in the intestinal tract – and absorbed into the circulation. These are thought to interact with natural male hormones to protect against benign prostatic hyperplasia, prostatitis and even prostate cancer.

This theory is strengthened by recent findings that blood

119

levels of dietary oestrogens are up to 110 times higher in Eastern races compared to inhabitants of the West.

There seems to be a paradox, however. Environmental oestrogens from other sources (e.g. PCBs, dioxins, traces of female HRT and oral contraceptive Pills in drinking water, bovine oestrogens in pregnant cows' milk) are currently implicated in the increased incidence of prostate cancer and the rapidly falling sperm counts observed in Western males *(see page 75)*.

How can environmental oestrogens protect Japanese men against prostate cancer yet seem to cause it in the West?

The answer seems to be that plant oestrogens (unlike synthetic environmental ones) are sufficiently similar to natural human oestrogens to trigger the production of a protein called Sex Hormone Binding Globulin (SHBG). This protein mops up the dietary oestrogens, as well as endogenous male hormones. Once hormones are bound to SHBG they are effectively inactivated. This reduces the prostate gland's overall exposure to hormones and therefore lowers the risk of prostate problems.

The plant oestrogens may also have a direct effect on male hormone production and metabolism, plus an effect on tumour cell growth.

Dietary Antioxidants

Eastern males eat many more yellow, orange, red and green vegetables (such as red, yellow and green peppers, broccoli, spinach, etc.) than Western males. These are high in the antioxidant vitamins E, C and betacarotene. By mopping up dangerous free radicals formed within the body during the normal processes of metabolism, they reduce the risk of coronary heart disease and cancer.

As in politics, a free radical is a highly unstable entity that races round picking fights and causing damage.

The molecular version carries a negative charge. It desperately tries to neutralize this by colliding with cell components and stealing a positive charge or off-loading its own negative one.

Each body cell is bombarded with an estimated 100,000 oxidation reactions every day – the number is twice as high in smokers.

If molecular DNA is damaged through these oxidations, errors can occur in gene sequences, or cancer-causing genes may be switched on. This increases the risk of all types of cancer, including that of the prostate gland.

A diet high in antioxidant vitamins and minerals protects against cancer (and coronary heart disease) by donating or accepting an unpaired electron to neutralize the free radical's negative charge before it can damage the cells.

Eastern males naturally obtain much higher amounts of these important antioxidant vitamins than Western males.

The National Cancer Institute (US) recommends a daily intake of at least 6 mg of betacarotene to decrease the risk of cancer. An intake of 15 mg per day is desirable – but this is only achievable by taking food supplements as well as paying attention to diet. Some experts in the UK also suggest we take daily dietary supplements of 150 mg vitamin C and 30–40 mg vitamin E.

Fibre

Vegetables are high in insoluble dietary fibre which stays in the intestinal tract and absorbs excess male hormones excreted in the bile. This helps flush them through the bowels so they are not reabsorbed to cause an imbalance.

Zinc

Vegetables are also rich in zinc, an important mineral for prostate health. Zinc forms part of an enzyme which switches on certain genes in response to hormone triggers and controls the sensitivity of prostate tissues to sex hormones. Intakes of at least 10 mg zinc per day are needed to maintain prostate health. (*See pages 364-5* for a list of foods that are rich in zinc.)

Dietary Saturated Fat

Latest research shows that men who follow a typical Western diet high in animal (saturated) fat have an increased risk of prostate cancer.

The more fat a man eats, the higher his risk of developing advanced prostate cancer. Saturated fat from red meat, mayonnaise, creamy salad dressings and butter seems to be most dangerous. There is no increased risk from any other dairy products such as milk or cheese.

Red meat is the food with the strongest positive link to advanced prostate disease. The researchers went so far as to recommend that males lower their intake of red meat if they want to reduce their risk of prostate cancer.

Instead, obtain essential fatty acids vital for prostate health such as linolenic and linoleic acids. Natural sources of these include nuts (e.g. walnuts) and seeds (e.g. pumpkin, sunflower; linseed). The WHO suggests that everyone should eat at least 30 g of nuts/seeds per day.

DIETARY TIPS TO DECREASE THE RISK OF PROSTATE CANCER

- Lose excess weight – fatty tissues secrete hormones and can trigger significant hormonal imbalances.
- Eat much less fat, especially saturated fat. Switch to low-fat milk, cheese, dressings etc. Fat intake should ideally be between 25–30 per cent of energy intake.
- Cut out red meat – or only eat it occasionally. Eat more skinless chicken and fish instead. Fish oil may have anti-cancer benefits.
- Eat at least a pound of fresh fruit or vegetables (not counting potatoes) every day. These should be raw or only lightly steamed. The WHO recommend a minimum of five portions of fresh fruit or vegetables per day.
- Try eating more Japanese-style foods – soy, rice, kohlrabi, Chinese leaves, etc.
- Eat plenty of whole grains, especially rye products.
- Eat more nuts and seeds – at least 30 g per day.

- Eat more fibre – 30–40 g per day.
- Increase your intake of unrefined carbohydrate (starchy foods) to the WHO recommendations of 50–70 per cent of energy intake.
- Perhaps take vitamin supplements to boost your diet:
  - vitamin E (30–40 mg)
  - vitamin C (around 150 mg)
  - betacarotene (around 15 mg)
- Perhaps take rye pollen extracts
- Perhaps take zinc supplements – up to 10 mg daily.

7

TESTOSTERONE AND MALE SEXUAL BEHAVIOUR

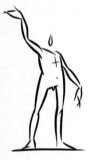

PUBERTY

Puberty is the stage between childhood and adulthood when secondary sexual characteristics develop, the sexual organs mature, and reproduction becomes possible. Emotional changes also occur and these, plus the physical changes of puberty, are referred to as adolescence.

In boys puberty usually starts between the ages of 10 and 14 years (although many hormonal changes can occur undetected before this time) and is complete by the age 15 to 17 years. It generally starts a year earlier in girls (age 9 to 13) when a good sign that puberty is in full swing is the appearance of the first menstrual bleed. In males, a similar stage of maturity is indicated by the occurrence of the first ejaculation. This often occurs at night, as a so-called 'wet dream'. This does not signify fertility, and is merely an indication that the testes have awakened and, together with the seminal vesicles and prostate gland, are starting their secretory function.

What triggers puberty is not fully understood. It may be due to the withdrawal of inhibitory nerve connections which damp down a part of the brain called the hypothalamus. Once this inhibition is removed, the hypothalamus releases pulses of a trigger substance called Leutinising Hormone-Releasing Hormone (LHRH). These LHRH pulses pass down nerve endings to stimulate the pituitary gland just beneath the hypothalamus, at the base of the brain.

The stimulated pituitary starts to secrete two other hormones which are essential for reproduction. These two hormones are Follicle Stimulating Hormone (FSH) and Leutinising Hormone (LH). FSH and LH enter the bloodstream and travel around the body to switch on the ovaries in females, or the testicles in males. FSH triggers the production and development of sperm, and LH triggers the production of the male hormone testosterone.

TESTOSTERONE AND ITS IMPORTANCE

Testosterone is the most important androgen, or male sex hormone. In males, 95 per cent is secreted by the testicles, with a small amount (5 per cent) also coming from the adrenal glands. A mature male secretes between 4 and 10 mg of testosterone per day. In females, small amounts of testosterone are also secreted by the adrenal glands and ovaries.

In each testis, the spaces between the convoluted seminiferous tubules (*see page 44*) are filled with nests of cells called the interstitial cells of Leydig. These contain fatty granules rich in cholesterol which are converted into testosterone through a series of chemical reactions. Testosterone is released into the bloodstream to stimulate the growth of bone and muscle, enlargement of the genitals and testicles, and sexual development. It is responsible for the male secondary sex characteristics that occur at puberty, and for sperm production.

The Effects of Testosterone Hormone

Testosterone hormone is responsible for:

125

- maintenance of male sex drive
- growth of the larynx and deepening of the voice
- growth of the penis, testes and scrotum
- development of rugged folds (rugae) in scrotal skin
- growth of the seminal vesicles and secretion of fluids rich in the sugar *fructose*
- growth of the prostate gland
- secretion of prostate fluids
- stimulation of sperm production
- maintenance of erectile/ejaculatory function
- fusion of bone ends (epiphyses)
- maintenance of muscle bulk.

Testosterone is broken down in the prostate gland and in hair follicles to form another hormone called dihydro-testosterone. This is twice as potent as testosterone and is thought to be responsible for:

- the growth of facial, armpit and limb hair
- maintenance of male-pattern pubic hair
- male pattern baldness
- acne
- benign enlargement of the prostate gland

The conversion of testosterone to dihydro-testosterone is controlled by an enzyme, 5-alpha-reductase. Males who lack this enzyme are genetically male, with normal functioning testicles, but are mistaken for girls until puberty. This is because their external genitals are sufficiently small and rudimentary to resemble those of the female. Once puberty starts, the presumed clitoris rapidly enlarges to become a penis and the 'labia' unfold to form a scrotum into which the testicles suddenly drop.

This defect is relatively common in a part of the Dominican Republic, where it is accepted as normal that a few of the little girls playing in the streets will grow up and turn into men. Those affected are known as 'guevedoces' meaning 'penis at twelves'.

These males seem to swop their psychosexual identity with no difficulty and, despite being reared as females, start functioning behaviourally as males. Interestingly, they do not develop acne, do not become bald and do not develop benign prostatic enlargement in later life.

These findings have helped researchers understand that it is dihydro-testosterone, and not testosterone, that may be responsible for male pattern baldness *(see page 239)* and benign prostatic enlargement *(see page 97)*.

PUBERTAL GROWTH SPURT

In boys, the peak growth spurt occurs between the ages of 12 and 17. This is controlled by both testosterone and growth hormone, with virtually every muscle and bone in the body affected. Differential growth in males means the shoulder girdle broadens more than the hips.

Changes also occur in body composition, so that lean body mass (muscle) increases while body fat percentage decreases so pubertal boys lose their chubbiness. The five stages of male genital development are indicated below. Ages given are the average for the onset of each stage:

Stage 1 pre-adolescence – penis, testes and scrotum of similar size and proportion as in early childhood

Stage 2 scrotum and testes enlarge; left testicle usually hangs lower than the right; the scrotum becomes baggier, slightly furrowed (rugose) and reddened; spermatogenesis begins (age 10–13)

Stage 3 testes and scrotum grow larger; penis first starts to lengthen, then becomes broader; sparse pubic hair develops; facial hair appears on upper lip and cheeks; body hair starts to appear on limbs and trunk (age 11–14)

Stage 4 further enlargement of testes and scrotum; scrotum darkens and becomes more furrowed; penis continues enlarging and glans starts to develop; pubic and body hair become more profuse, with hair growing around the base of the penis; major growth spurt occurs (age 13–17)

THE COMPLETE BOOK OF MEN'S HEALTH

Stage 5 adult stage, with genitals fully matured; pubic hair extends up the abdominal midline in male pattern; facial hair extends to lower lip and chin (age 17–18)

Breaking Voice

Testosterone causes the male voice box (larynx) to enlarge and the vocal cords to become longer and thicker. This causes the pitch of the voice to drop; this deepening of the voice is often referred to as the voice 'breaking'. This tends to occur around the age of 14, but the majority of boys do not notice it is happening as the changes are gradual. Some boys notice a tight feeling in their throat which passes after a few weeks, and may be accompanied by a croaky voice. This is nothing to worry about.

MALE SEXUAL BEHAVIOUR

In human males, sexual behaviour is dependent on testosterone hormone. This produces increased sexual interest and sex drive and intensifies innate patterns of sexual behaviour. Giving testosterone to heterosexuals increases their interest in the opposite sex, and the administration of testosterone to homosexual males intensifies their homosexual drive – it does not convert it into a heterosexual one.

In a study of over 4,000 American men it was found that husbands with high testosterone levels were 43 per cent more likely to get divorced and 38 per cent more likely to have extramarital affairs than men with lower levels. They were also 50 per cent less likely to get married in the first place.

Men with the lowest testosterone levels were more likely to get married and to stay married successfully. This may be because low testosterone levels make men more docile, less aggressive, better humoured and more home loving.

Interestingly, testosterone levels seem to affect the career a man will follow. Those with highest testosterone levels are likely to become athletes, actors and entertainers – professions that are associated with competitive, aggressive or extrovert behaviour.

Some chemicals have an anti-testosterone action and are called anti-androgens. The administration of cyproterone acetate or medroxyprogesterone acetate can decrease the male sex drive and interfere with the ability to produce an erection. These drugs are sometimes used to treat sex offenders.

Castration (removal of the testes) is eventually followed by a reduction in sexual activity, but this may not be for several years. In many cases, sexual activity does not peter out altogether. This may be due to an increased output of testosterone from the adrenal glands, which usually only provide 5 per cent of circulating testosterone levels.

In males who do lose their sex drive and ability to have erections, treatment with testosterone replacement effectively reverses these changes and restores sexual activity to its former level.

What Is A Normal Sex Drive?

According to various surveys, 40 per cent of British couples make love more than three times per week, 35 per cent make love once or twice a week and 15 per cent make love two to three times per month. Nine per cent of couples make love less than this or not at all.

The National Survey of Sexual Attitudes and Lifestyles in the UK (published in 1994) found that men aged 25–34 years of age made love around five times per month. As age rose to 55–59 years, levels of activity fell to twice per month.

According to The *Esquire* Survey (1992) of 800 men, 2 per cent of males have sex once a day or more and 11 per cent have sex four to six times per week. The most common frequency seems to be two to three times per week. Only 5 per cent of non-virgin males were not actively indulging in sexual relationships.

The duration of a relationship is also significant. Other

129

surveys have found that over 50 per cent of couples together for under three years make love more than three times per week. After four or more years together, only 25 per cent maintain this frequency.

Aphrodisiacs

A number of aphrodisiacs have proved popular over the ages. Most derive from obviously phallic articles. The association of powdered rhinoceros horn and bananas with hardness and virility is easy to see, but feasting on the still warm brains of recently decapitated criminals seems eccentric – until you realize that erection is a common side-effect of sudden spinal trauma. This is known rather cruelly as 'Custer's Last Stand'. Safer reputed aphrodisiacs include oysters, champagne, ginseng, *Eleutherococcus* (Siberian ginseng) and, surprisingly, raspberries.

Pheromones

Pheromones are volatile chemicals that are secreted in very small amounts in our skin oils. They are mostly undetectable at a conscious level but have powerful effects on mood. Pheromones are thought to be the key to human sexual attraction, and recently the first one to be isolated (from skin fragments within a discarded orthopaedic plaster cast) was studied for its effects. Liquid concentrates of this human pheromone were tested on 40 volunteers, and feelings described as 'a contented high' put pheromone recipients into a friendly, responsive mood. Extracts may be added to aftershave and skin perfumes in the near future, perhaps with devastating effects.

THE MALE MENOPAUSE

It now seems certain that some males experience a form of male menopause, or *viripause*. Testosterone is secreted continuously in the male and, unlike the female sex hormone oestrogen, does not peak and fall in a monthly cycle. Highest blood levels occur during the teens and early twenties and gradually fall off thereafter.

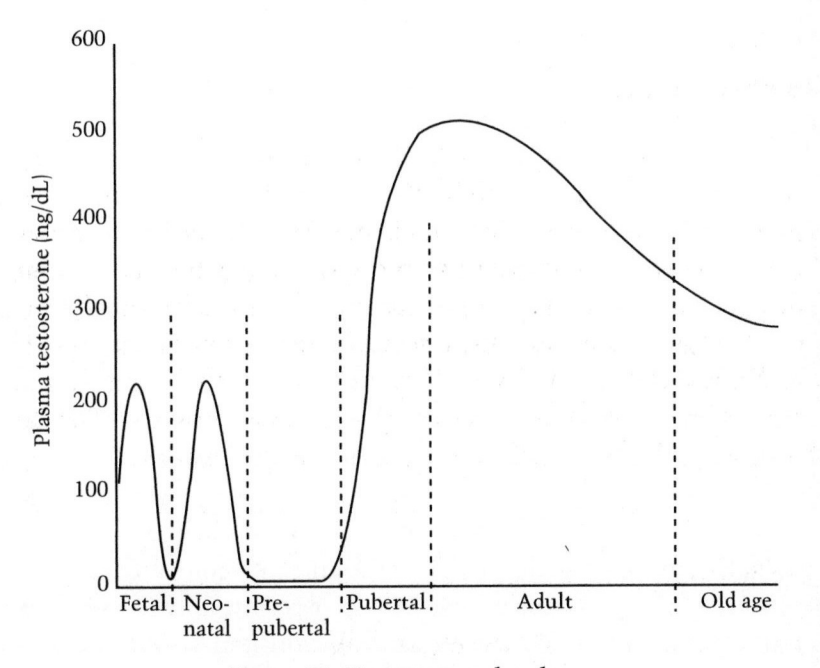

Figure 17: Testosterone levels

During middle age, circulating levels of testosterone fall slightly and, in some males, symptoms of tiredness, irritability, lowered libido, aching joints, dry skin, insomnia, excessive sweating, hot flushes and depression are triggered. In the long term, bone thinning (osteoporosis) may occur in a similar manner to that affecting post-menopausal women. Between the ages of 40 and 70 years, male bone density falls by up to 15 per cent, and men also lose an average of 5–10 kg in muscle weight. Sperm counts tend to drop and erectile failure occurs more frequently – all evidence that testosterone hormone is failing to do its job.

Many men with these symptoms have a testosterone level within the normal range, however. Their symptoms may therefore be due to an interaction problem between testosterone and its receptors, or to excessive alcohol intake *(see page 272)* or stress levels *(see page 283)*, both of which increase the rate of testosterone turnover. Another possibility is that the levels of circulating Sex Hormone Binding Globulin (SHBG) are high. This protein mops up free testosterone and binds it in an inactive form. This would explain why the testosterone is present and measurable in the bloodstream, yet cannot exert its usual effects.

Male hormone replacement therapy (HRT) for male menopausal symptoms involves administering testosterone pills up to three times per day for three to six months. Alternatively, an implant is inserted into the buttock which will slowly release testosterone over a six-month period.

Treatment is aimed at raising testosterone levels to normal – not to excessively high levels – and will not turn a man into a sexual dynamo. It merely restores whatever level of libido is normal for any particular male. Those who have received treatment claim to feel better within two weeks, with increased energy, better moods and a renewed interest in sex.

Male HRT is still controversial and not many doctors will prescribe it. Increased levels of testosterone have been linked with cancer of the prostate gland. If you feel you need further assessment, most doctors will be happy to refer you on to a hormone specialist (endocrinologist).

Non-hormonal ways of beating the male menopause include:

- stopping smoking
- drinking less alcohol
- losing excess weight
- taking more exercise
- cutting down on caffeine intake
- taking a multinutrient supplement (deficiencies of vitamins and minerals can exacerbate hormonal imbalances)
- checking that symptoms are not caused by other prescribed medications
- seeking counselling for relationship or sexual difficulties.

MASTURBATION

Masturbation is now accepted as a natural, healthy activity. Surveys reveal that 80 per cent of men masturbate regularly: 13 per cent of males do it more than three times per week, 25 per cent do it one to three times per week and 15 per cent masturbate two or three times per month. Men who are not sexually active and who do not masturbate will eventually experience a 'wet dream' – a nocturnal emission of semen.

Masturbation is only harmful if it causes feelings of guilt and encourages furtiveness. Tales of masturbation causing ill effects such as excessive hair, visual impairment or physical deformity are the products of repressed minds and have no basis in reality.

HOMOSEXUALITY

The evolution of human sexual behaviour is complex. It involves instinct, developmental factors, possibly a genetic component, social pressures and the availability of partners of the preferred sex.

It is frequently claimed that 10 per cent of males have homosexual tendencies, but this is probably an underestimate. If those who experimented with homosexuality during adolescence were included, this figure would be higher.

Kinsey, one of the first sexologists, found that 37 per cent of males in his studies admitted to experiencing at least one homosexual encounter to the point of orgasm. Another study involving almost 3,000 college males aged 18–25 years found the equivalent figure was 30 per cent. Even these high figures may be underestimates, as sexual questionnaires are notorious for eliciting untruths.

The 1994 UK National Survey of Sexual Attitudes and Lifestyles found that 6 per cent of 8,000 males reported some kind of homosexual experience, of which 3.6 per cent was genital contact with another man. Only 1.4 per cent had had a male sexual partner within the previous two years, a figure that seems extraordinarily low.

133

Homosexuality consists of a spectrum of behaviour:

- predominantly heterosexual with incidental homosexual experiences
- equally heterosexual and homosexual
- predominantly homosexual with incidental heterosexual experiences or
- exclusively homosexual.

Sexual tendency and preference may not always match observed sexual activity, however, as the high prevalence of homosexual behaviour within prisons demonstrates. Equally, social pressures may drive a man with a strong homosexual drive to remain exclusively heterosexual throughout his life.

Several theories suggest that homosexuality is a biological phenomenon with a physiological basis. For example, some men may have hormone receptors that only partially respond to circulating sex hormones. This might result in a lack of the hormone-dependent desire to seek a partner of the opposite sex for procreation.

Recent research suggests that some centres in the brain are responsible for sexual behaviour. The male behaviour centre, which contains androgen receptors, is in the anterior hypo-thalamic area of the brain. The female centre is in an area called the ventromedial nuclear region of the brain. These centres are thought to develop according to the levels of circulating sex hormones during early foetal life. This response is in turn dependent on the successful interaction of a sex hormone and its equivalent receptors. It seems logical that differences in the responsiveness of receptors in these areas might result in homosexual as opposed to heterosexual behaviour.

This theory was recently strengthened by the finding that an area in the anterior hypothalamus in homosexual men has the anatomical form usually found in women rather than the structure typical of heterosexual males. The cluster of cells involved (INAH-3) is on average smaller in gay men (and the same size as the cluster in women), while another area, the suprachiasmatic nucleus, is twice as large.

It is not that simple, however. Some gay men have an INAH-3 nucleus which is the same size as heterosexual males and, in any case, size differences are small and may be subject to measurement errors. Further research also suggests that the cables of nerves connecting the left- and right-hand sides of the brain are larger in gay men than in heterosexuals.

Studies with 28 pairs of male twins show that if one identical twin is gay, the other twin is three times more likely to be gay than if the twins are non-identical. This suggests a genetic component. Scientists believe the next step will be the identification of the specific genes that influence homosexual behaviour – one has apparently already been traced in the Drosophila (fruit fly).

Whether or not these brain or genetic structural difference are linked with homosexuality is as yet unknown. If they are, it would imply that sexuality varies genetically, in the same way that some people are left-handed, others right-handed and some ambidextrous.

TRANSSEXUALISM

A few males suffer from *gender dysphoria*, in which they feel varying degrees of discomfort with their biological sex from early childhood. Occasionally, this is a stress-related phenomenon.

Transvestitism is a very mild form of gender dysphoria and is limited to a desire to wear clothing usually reserved for the opposite (in this case female) sex. This produces feelings of calm and rightness which others can find difficult to understand.

Some men feel they are trapped in the wrong body and have an overwhelming desire to lose all external evidence of manhood and to become anatomical females.

Sex change operations are available for transsexuals but are only undertaken after extensive counselling. Usually, males requesting a sex change operation must first demonstrate that they can live and function as a woman for an extended time prior to the operation. This may involve the trauma of being disowned by family, friends and even children. In addition, the operative complications and the side-effects of the necessary drugs can be serious.

Without proper preparation for life in the opposite gender, an unattainable rosy fantasy of what it would be like can result, after the operation, in severe disappointment, depression, suicide or an impossible request to reverse the complex surgery undertaken. In appropriately chosen cases, however, gender reassignment transforms the quality of life.

In male-to-female gender reassignments, the first stage is to take female hormones by mouth – these will be continued for life. This encourages the breasts to enlarge and feminizes the skin. Unwanted hair is removed by electrolysis and, if male pattern baldness is present, a wig is worn. Sometimes the breasts are enlarged with surgical implants.

The next stage involves removal of the penis and testes plus fashioning of a functional vagina. In some cases the vagina is fashioned from a length of large bowel (colon) which is then stitched in place. This procedure has the advantage of producing a moist vagina that secretes mucus.

Another approach is to retain the skin of the penis and glans and to fashion the vagina from these. This has the advantage of leaving some of the nerves intact so that some sexual pleasure is still possible, but lubrication must be added for intercourse.

During the operation, the urethra is identified and protected by passing a catheter into the bladder. The spongy tissues of the penis are then carefully dissected away from the skin and urethra and discarded. The remaining skin is then pulled down and inverted so that it is pushed up into the pelvis where the root of the penis used to lie. The scrotal skin is used to fashion artificial vaginal lips (labia) and the urethra is shortened and stitched into place in front of the new vagina. After the operation, vaginal dilators are needed to maintain vaginal size and stop the skin contracting down.

8

MALE SEXUAL DYSFUNCTION

IMPOTENCE

The word impotence is derived from the Latin *impotentia*, meaning *lack of power*. It was first used to describe loss of sexual power in 1655 in, of all places, a treatise entitled 'Church History of Britain' by Thomas Fuller.

Impotence is the inability to obtain or maintain an erection for the satisfactory completion of heterosexual vaginal intercourse. Satisfactory is usually taken to mean an adequate erection, of sufficient hardness, maintained for a sufficient length of time, that ends in a controlled ejaculation and provides sexual satisfaction for both partners.

Impotence is a common and distressing condition affecting 10 to 30 per cent of men on a regular basis. All age groups are involved, but due to embarrassment or a mistaken belief that nothing can be done, victims often suffer in silence and despair. Whatever the cause of impotence, 99 per cent of men can get their erections back by one of the many treatment options now available.

It is often assumed that impotence is a purely psychological problem, but in 40 per cent of cases a physical cause is involved. If a man awakes with a morning erection or can masturbate to orgasm when alone, the problem is more likely to be psychological rather than physical.

If a male never manages an erection, even on waking, a physical problem is likely and this must be carefully looked into by a doctor specializing in urology.

During a night's sleep, between four and eight erections occur naturally unless there is a physical blockage preventing them. A special device can be attached to the penis before going to sleep that regularly measures penile diameter and rigidity throughout the night. This is useful for differentiating between physical and psychological causes of impotence.

Often, however, both physical and psychological factors play a role as a vicious circle builds up that causes anxiety and negative feelings to set in.

Physical Causes of Impotence

The most common physical cause of impotence is tiredness, overwork and stress. It is perfectly normal to perform under par in these circumstances. Other physical causes include drug side-effects, hardening of the arteries (atherosclerosis), leaking valves that stop blood pooling within spongy tissues, fibrosis, hormonal imbalances and nerve damage.

Drug Side-effects

Drug side-effects are a common and reversible cause of impotence. Among the prescribable drugs, the worst offenders are beta-blockers – which work by damping down the activity of certain types of nerve. Beta-blockers are excellent drugs which are frequently prescribed to treat high blood pressure, angina, heart attacks, anxiety, palpitations, migraine, glaucoma and an over-active thyroid, but if this side-effect becomes troublesome it is important to tell your doctor so you can be switched to a different type of drug.

Thiazide diuretics (water tablets) prescribed to lower high

blood pressure or reduce fluid accumulation in the body can also trigger erectile failure. Patients taking diuretics are twice as likely to be impotent as those on no drugs. Again, tell your doctor; alternative treatments are available.

Anti-depressant tablets affect nerve endings in the nervous system and can also be at fault.

If you are taking any drugs at all it is worth asking your doctor or a pharmacist whether these are likely to affect your sex drive.

It is easy to forget that cigarette smoke contains a powerful drug, nicotine. Cigarette smoking is closely linked with erectile failure, and there is a clear dose-related effect: the more cigarettes smoked per day, the less rigid the erection. Cigarette smoking damages blood vessels and hastens 'furring up' of the arteries.

Atherosclerosis

Hardening and furring of the arteries is common in late middle age. Sometimes, the arteries leading to the penis become blocked and furred up with cholesterol deposits. This poor circulation means blood cannot flow into the penis in the volume required for a normal erection, and impotence results.

Tests that outline blood flow into the penis (using dyes that show up on X-ray) will show any narrowing of the arteries that may be the cause. Ultrasound is also sometimes used to measure changes to the blood flow after injection with an erection-inducing drug.

Slow Leaks

In some males, erection starts off rigidly and then slowly sags due to a slow leak of blood out of the corpora cavernosa and corpus spongiosum (*see pages 3 and 4*). This is due to a weakness in the mechanisms that constrict outlet veins and prevent pooling blood from draining away during erection. This problem can be detected by special tests using dyes that show up on X-ray (cavernosometry). Venous leaks are a common cause of impotence in older men. Some men suffer from both poor blood supply and a venous leak.

Fibrosis

If the blood supply is normal, fibrosis or a build-up of scar tissue (e.g. Peyronie's Disease, *see page 15*) can make the penis rigid on one side, rather than expansile. This stops the penis inflating fully, or makes it curve dramatically and painfully to one side. This can cause partial or total impotence. Surgical treatment to remove the scar tissue, or to take a tuck in the opposite side so erections become straight again, can help solve this problem.

Hormonal Imbalances

Occasionally, an hormonal imbalance may be the cause of impotence, especially if testosterone hormone levels are too low or prolactin hormone levels too high. If you suffer from impotence you will have blood tests to screen for hormonal problems. If an imbalance is found, this is usually easily treated once its cause is sorted out.

Diabetes

Diabetes causes impotence for two main reasons: it encourages furring up of the arteries (atherosclerosis) and, if not well controlled, can lead to permanent nerve damage from the high levels of circulating sugar.

Nerve Damage

Diseases or injuries that affect the nerves can cause impotence. This includes men who suffer from severe multiple sclerosis, or who have sustained a spinal cord injury as a result, for example, of breaking their back. Sometimes reflex erections occur but ejaculation is not normally possible without electrical stimulation.

The Treatment of Physical Impotence

The treatment of physical impotence is now sophisticated. Several options are available after full investigations have suggested the likely cause.

Oral Drugs

International trials of an oral drug treatment for impotence are currently under way. The drug, a derivative of yohimbine hydrochloride, is derived from the African *Pausinystalis yohimbe* tree. Results of the trials are expected soon but it will be a few years before it becomes widely available on the market.

Viagra

Viagra (Sildenafil citrate) is the first oral drug to become available for the treatment of male impotence. It is taken around an hour before sexual activity and helps three out of four men with erectile difficulties maintain an erection. It works by blocking certain receptors (Type 5 phosphodiesterase receptors) in the penis. This relaxes smooth muscle fibres in blood vessels leading to the penis, as well as in the spongy tissues (corpora cavernosa) of the penis itself so that more blood arrives in the area and pools in the spongy tissues to produce an erection. It is not an aphrodisiac and will only trigger an erection in men who have a healthy sex drive and who are sexually stimulated.

Viagra can help men with impotence linked with both physical and psychological causes including diabetes, high blood pressure, depression, spinal cord injury and prostate surgery. In clinical trials, 70 to 90 per cent of men with impotence (aged 34 – 70 years) reported an improvement in the quality of their erections, compared with only around a quarter of those taking inactive placebo. This effect was independently confirmed by the men's partners. Viagra is well tolerated and the most common side-effects include headache, nasal congestion,

141

indigestion, flushing and pelvic muscle pain. Around 3 per cent of patients experience mild, occasional changes in colour vision and light sensitivity. There have been reports of users suffering from heart attacks, but this may partly be related to the fact that those needing it are more likely to be unfit, middle-aged or elderly males with conditions such as diabetes, high blood pressure or hardening and furring up of the arteries which caused their impotence in the first place. It should not be taken by men taking other blood vessel dilation drugs (such as nitrates used to treat angina) as this may lead to a sudden and potentially serious drop in blood pressure.

MUSE

MUSE – which stands for Medicated Urethral System for Erection – is another new approach to treating male impotence. Rather than injecting the drug alprostadil into the penis (as with P.I.P.E., page 143), a special delivery device allows a pellet the size of a grain of rice to be inserted painlessly into the opening of the urinary tube (urethra) at the tip of the penis. Alprostadil works by relaxing muscle fibres and dilating blood vessels in the penis so more blood flows into the area. Erection usually follows within five to ten minutes and lasts from 30 – 60 minutes. MUSE is effective in almost 70 per cent of men using it. Few side-effects occur and almost 90 per cent of men using it rate MUSE as 'very comfortable', 'comfortable' or 'neutral' to use and preferable to injection into the penis. MUSE is inserted as follows:

- After urination, lie down, stretch the penis to its full length and slowly insert the stem of the MUSE delivery system into the end of the penis.
- Press the ejector button to release the pellet into the penis.
- Slowly and gently rock the applicator to and fro to make sure the medication separates from the tip of the applicator.
- After withdrawing the applicator, either you or your partner should then roll the penis between your hands for 10 seconds to distribute the medication along the urethra.

No more than two doses should be used in any 24-hour period. If your partner is pregnant, MUSE should only be used together with a condom.

Topical GTN

Glyceryl trinitrate (GTN) is a drug normally used to treat heart angina pains. GTN dilates blood vessels and increases blood flow. Research has found that GTN patches applied to the penis for one to two hours before intercourse can help to overcome impotence. Of 10 males aged 45–71 who had suffered impotence for an average of five years, four achieved an erection with intercourse and ejaculation – a success rate of 40 per cent.

The use of GTN patches has an advantage over GTN creams, as the latter are absorbed by vaginal tissues and cause the side-effect of headaches in any female partners.

Vacuum Erections

For a vacuum erection the penis is placed in a plastic cylinder from which air is extracted via a pump. The resultant partial vacuum makes the penis fill with blood and triggers an erection. A tight ring is then placed around the base of the penile shaft to trap the blood and maintain rigidity. The penis then remains erect once the vacuum cylinder is removed. Obviously, as it acts rather like a tourniquet, the penis looks a little blue, and the ring can only be left in place for a short while (otherwise the blood supply of the penis may be compromised). Another problem is that the elastic band prevents semen coming out of the tip of the penis during ejaculation. Semen may seep out later, or may wash into the bladder to be urinated away. This is not harmful but does affect fertility.

P.I.P.E.

Some patients are taught to give themselves an injection into the shaft of the penis. This is known as P.I.P.E. – Pharmacologically Induced Penile Erection. The injections are given via a very fine needle inserted into the corpora cavernosa. The shaft of the penis is not very pain-sensitive and the injections are described as no more painful than a mosquito bite. After withdrawing the needle, the injection site is pressed firmly for 30 seconds so that no bleeding occurs. After 5–10 minutes, an erection starts to form as the arteries supplying blood to the penis dilate and draining veins constrict.

The commonly used drug, papaverine, can induce prolonged erections and priapism *(see page 16)*, however. Priapism is a surgical emergency – the penis needs to be drained of trapped blood to restore the circulation. Papaverine can also cause internal scarring and curvature (Peyronie's disease) in a few males. In the majority of cases, nevertheless, P.I.P.E. is very successful and has transformed the lives of many impotent males.

Another drug, prostaglandin E1, is prescribed instead of papaverine by some doctors as it has a lower risk of side-effects.

A new development is a self-injection system known as Caverject (alprostadil). This works in a similar manner to prostaglandin E1 and can be prescribed by doctors. Some men find it more painful than other drug treatments, however.

Vascular Surgery

If there is a physical blockage to penile blood inflow, it is possible to have an arterial by-pass graft operation in which the blockage is by-passed using a length of vein, or synthetic tubing. In some cases, a single stricture can be dilated with a special balloon inserted into the artery under X-ray control.

Another successful approach is to hook up another artery, which normally delivers blood to the lower abdominal muscles, to the penis. This is joined to one of the penile arteries using microsurgical techniques; the procedure instantly increases the blood flow to the penis. The lower abdominal muscles do not suffer either, as several other arteries also supply them with blood. Some of the penile-draining veins are usually tied off at the same time to increase the effect: this combines a better blood flow coming in with a weaker blood flow draining out. Success rates are as high as 70 per cent.

Arterial by-pass surgery involves a fairly large incision extending up the lower abdomen, and requires a stay of several days in hospital.

If impotence is due solely to a slow venous leak, this is simply corrected by tying off the major veins draining the penis. This procedure is known as venous ligation, and is successful in 50 per cent of cases. Occasionally, new veins open up after the operation and venous leaking may recur after a few years.

Surgical Implants

Prostheses are devices that can be surgically implanted into the penis to produce erection. There are two main types:

1. semi-rigid rods giving the patient half an erection all of the time
2. complicated, inflatable devices with small pumps implanted in the scrotum and a fluid reservoir bag implanted in the abdomen or pelvis. These devices are activated by squeezing the pump or activating a trigger button in the scrotum. Deflation is brought about by pressing another button.

Some semi-rigid implants have an embedded silver wire to make them bendable. The penis can then be bent and 'parked' when not in use. Newer designs consist of implanted, inter-locking discs made of plastic. These can be rotated in one direction to lock and become rigid, then, after intercourse, rotated the other way to become flaccid when not required.

Insertion of an implant takes from one to three hours, depending on the type selected. The procedure is done under a local anaesthetic, or under a spinal epidural (the body is numbed from the waist down).

It takes around two weeks for the discomfort and swelling of the operation to settle down, especially under the scrotum where the base of the penis is situated. Intercourse can be resumed from four to six weeks after the operation, depending on the procedure used. The main risk with penile implantation is post-operative infection, but this seems to be relatively rare.

Ninety per cent of men with an implant are entirely happy with its performance. Most implants are invisible, although the semi-rigid rods can make the penis stick out a little bit at all times. This does not look abnormal, however.

Herbal Remedies that can Overcome Impotence

CATUABA

Extracts from the bark of a Brazilian tree, Catuaba (*Erythroxylon catuaba*) are one of the most successful prosexual herbs for males. Catuaba is known locally as the Tree of Togetherness and a famous Brazilian saying states: 'Until a father reaches 60, the son is his; after that the son is Catuaba's' – for the supplement is widely used to maintain potency and fertility in older males and to treat male impotence. Catuaba acts as an aphrodisiac, promoting erotic dreams and increased sexual energy. Erotic dreams usually start within five to 21 days of taking extracts regularly, followed by increased sexual desire. It also improves peripheral blood flow, which may be another mechanism of action in boosting sexual performance, and has been used to combat extreme exhaustion.

Dose

1 gram on waking, and 1 g on going to bed. There is no evidence of unwanted side-effects, even after long-term use.

DAMIANA

Extracts from the leaves of a small shrub, Damiana (*Turnera diffusa aphrodisiaca*) have a prosexual action due to its volatile oils. These have a gentle, irritant effect on the genitals to produce tingling and throbbing plus increased blood flow to the penis. These combined effects increase sexual desire, enhance sexual pleasure and stimulate sexual performance. When drunk as a tea, it produces a mild euphoria and some people use it almost as a recreational drug. It is particularly useful where anxiety and depression contribute to low sex drive, impotence or premature ejaculation.

Dose
Dried herb: 1 – 4 g three times a day.
Capsules: 200 – 800 mg daily.

Usually taken on an occasional basis when needed rather than regularly. No serious side-effects reported. May reduce iron absorption from the gut, so should not be used long term.

GINKGO

Extracts from the leaves of the Ginkgo biloba, or Maidenhair tree, are widely used to improve blood flow to the brain and boost memory. It is less widely known that ginkgo also relaxes blood vessels in the genitals and that it is a true prosexual herbal supplement. It has been shown to improve blood flow to the penis and improve erections even at a relatively low dose. A beneficial effect is usually noticed after six to eight weeks' treatment in men with erectile dysfunction; half of impotent males taking it had regained full potency after six months. In a study where 50 men took ginkgo for nine months, all those who had previously relied on injectable drugs to achieve an erection regained their potency. Of the 30 men who were not helped by medical drugs, 19 achieved erections with ginkgo.

Dose
Extracts standardized for at least 24 per cent ginkgolides: 40 – 60 mg two to three times a day (take a minimum of 120 mg daily). Stimulating effects last from three – six hours, but effects may not be noticed until after 10 days' treatment.

GINSENG

Ginseng (*Panax ginseng; P quinquefolium*) is a well-known herbal supplement used as a revitalizing tonic and to overcome stress. It contains several plant hormones that have an aphrodisiac action and improve erections. Recent research suggests it works in a similar way to Viagra (Sildenafil citrate) by increasing blood flow to the penis. In one study, men with impotence where given either Korean red ginseng or inactive placebo for 60 days. Frequency of sexual intercourse, morning erection, firmness of penis and size of tumescence were significantly greater (67 per cent) in those taking the ginseng than those taking placebo (28 per cent).

Dose

Choose a standardized product, preferably with a content of at least 5 per cent ginsenosides for American ginseng and 15 per cent ginsenosides for Korean ginseng. Start with a low dose and work up from 200 – 1,000 mg per day. Most people find 600 mg daily is effective without being too stimulating. If you find Chinese ginseng too stimulating, however, you could try American ginseng which seems to have a more gentle action. Best taken in a two-weeks-on, two-weeks-off cycle – do not take for more than six weeks without a break. Ginseng should not be used by men with high blood pressure or glaucoma. It is best to avoid taking other stimulants such as caffeine containing products and drinks while taking ginseng.

MUIRA PUAMA (*PTYCHOPETALUM OLACOIDES*)

Extracts from the roots and bark of a Brazilian tree, Muira Puama – popularly known as Potency Wood – are effective for boosting low sex drive and overcoming many cases of impotence. It is thought to work through a direct action on brain chemicals, by stimulating nerve endings in the genitals and by boosting the function of sex hormones, especially testosterone. It has a 'dynamic' effect in over 60 per cent of men complaining of lack of sexual and over 50 per cent of those with erectile dysfunction felt it was of benefit.

Dose

1 – 1.5 g daily for two weeks. No serious side-effects have been reported at therapeutic doses.

For further information on Viagra, herbal remedies and other impotence treatments, see *Increase Your Sex Drive* by Dr Sarah Brewer (published by Thorsons).

Psychological Causes of Impotence

Psychological problems account for 60 per cent of cases of impotence. Counselling and psychotherapy are helpful and often result in dramatic improvement.

Psychological problems are usually based on fear, guilt or feelings of inadequacy. The more a man worries about not getting an erection, the more the erection is likely to fail. It becomes a self-fulfilling prophecy. Relaxation training and professional psychosexual counselling are vital.

Psychosexual counselling often involves a temporary ban on penetrative sex. Sufferers are taught to relax with their partner while exploring each other's bodies afresh. Usually, it is agreed in advance that even if an erection is achieved, sexual penetration will not be attempted.

After several weeks of abstinence, couples are then allowed to try having sex with the partner on top. This is known as the Mistress position. The so-called 'Missionary position' (man on top) is not good for men with semi-rigid erections.

A caring and sympathetic partner is important. He or she is an invaluable support during the investigation and treatment of the partner's impotence. A partner who mocks or ridicules (or even feels overly sorry for) a man's performance is making the problem worse and may even have contributed to it in the first place.

PREMATURE EJACULATION

Premature ejaculation is the most common male sexual dysfunction. There are three different ways of defining it:

1. if the man comes before he wants to or before his partner wants him to
2. if ejaculation occurs before the penis penetrates the vagina
3. if the man cannot stop himself ejaculating for at least one minute after penetrating his partner.

149

Most men experience premature ejaculation several times during their lives – most commonly when losing their virginity. It also occurs in over 50 per cent of males when making love to a new partner for the first time. Premature ejaculation is particularly common among teenagers and tends to become less of a problem for men in their twenties and thirties and beyond.

If a man can stop ejaculating for anything over one minute after penetration, this is normal. It may not sound very long, but our primitive male ancestors were originally designed to thrust only five or six times before reaching orgasm. Humans are unique among the animal kingdom in using sex for pleasure. The male chimpanzee, for example, ejaculates within 30 seconds of intercourse and the female satisfies herself by mating with many males in quick succession.

Premature ejaculation is usually due to anxiety – especially if a new partner is involved. This often results in eagerness and over-excitement. The other main cause is anxiety about performance – whether you will be 'good enough' for your partner or will fail to satisfy. No man wants to feel his performance is not up to scratch.

Other causes of premature ejaculation are the man feeling that his partner is not really interested in sex, or if either partner has difficulty in showing or responding to affection.

Sometimes the opposite problem of retarded ejaculation occurs – especially if the male is trying to postpone his orgasm to make sure his partner is satisfied (see below).

The easiest way to make premature ejaculation less of a problem is to bring your partner to the point of orgasm during foreplay. Then, when your partner is about to come, penetration can occur or you can wait until after your partner's orgasm before entering. There are eight other techniques that help to overcome premature ejaculation. As some of these seem to take the pleasure out of sex, they will not suit every man:

1. Wear a condom. This damps down sensory stimulation and usually helps to prolong intercourse.
2. Use a local anaesthetic cream to numb the tip of the penis.

These creams can be bought over the counter. Make sure you buy a pure anaesthetic cream rather than a preparation intended for piles, as the latter sometimes contains other agents that might cause irritation to both yourself and your partner.

3. Tense the buttock muscles while thrusting. This helps to mask signals from nerve endings in the penis and gives you something else to concentrate on.

4. Think about something other than sex while making love, such as problems at work, or your plans for the following day. By taking your mind off sex (just for a moment!) you may find you can penetrate your partner for longer.

5. Just before ejaculation, the testicles naturally rise in the scrotum to sit close to the base of the penis. If you gently pull the testicles back down into the scrotum, you may find this helps delay ejaculation. Be careful not to twist them, however.

6. If you are able to penetrate your partner, pre-arrange a signal, such as saying 'stop'. Then, when you feel you are about to come, both you and your partner can become still and stop thrusting. This may help to prolong intercourse and can be repeated as often as necessary.

7. The most famous way of preventing premature ejaculation is the 'squeeze' technique. The man's partner gently masturbates him until he says he is about to come. The partner then gently squeezes the penis between the thumb and two fingers just below the helmet, where the glans joins the shaft. The squeeze should be firmly sustained for about five seconds and then the pressure relaxed for a minute. This can be repeated to postpone ejaculation as often as you wish and is often highly successful. By retraining your sexual habits, you will eventually be able to achieve normal intercourse. During intercourse, a man can also squeeze his penis himself, providing he has enough prior warning of impending ejaculation to reach down in time.

8. After experiencing premature ejaculation, wait for an hour and then try again. The second erection often lasts longer and orgasm can be delayed.

If none of these tips work, seek help from your doctor. You can be referred for professional psychosexual counselling in which you and your partner will be given help and exercises to try. Often, intercourse and orgasm are banned altogether, which takes away the pressure to perform.

Retarded Ejaculation

Retarded ejaculation is the inability of a man to ejaculate, despite having prolonged intercourse, adequate stimulation, and an intense desire to do so. This is an occasional occurrence in most men, especially when tired, but some males have never achieved ejaculation during sexual intercourse. Most affected men are able to ejaculate during masturbation.

Medical conditions such as diabetes, an enlarged prostate gland, previous prostate operation or certain drugs (e.g. water tablets, tricyclic antidepressants, treatment for high blood pressure) are sometimes at fault.

The commonest cause of ejaculatory failure, however, are psychological inhibitions such as in the case of:

- newlyweds sleeping next door to their parents
- discovering a spouse is unfaithful
- a recent condom break when pregnancy would have been disastrous
- having recently been interrupted during sex, such as by your children.

These episodes can trigger retarded ejaculation through a sub-conscious inhibition of the ejaculatory reflex. Make sure your surroundings are compatible with unstressful sex – that is, quiet, with no risk of interruption or being overheard, warm and comfortable. If problems persist you can be referred for psychotherapy, which will involve a structured programme of sexual exercises as 'homework'.

9

CONTRACEPTION

Contraception is now as much men's responsibility as it is women's.

At present the only contraceptive practices that involve a personal decision by the man are:

- the withdrawal method
- the male condom
- vasectomy.

This situation is likely to change over the next few years, however. Egyptian doctors have perfected The Jockstrap *(see page 68)*, which stops sperm production through a combination of increased heat and an electrostatic field across the testes. A male hormonal contraceptive injection could be available within two years, and a male Pill is actively being researched.

The gene complex responsible for switching on spermatogenesis has also just been identified and is known as the *azoospermia factor*. It is sited on the male Y chromosome, and mutations or deletions in this spot are linked with male infertility. Switching this gene off would theoretically lead to a future method of male contraception.

The Durex Report (1994) questioned 12,600 people about

their attitudes to sex and contraception. The main contraceptive relied on by almost one in four couples was the condom, with around one in five favouring the oral contraceptive Pill:

MAIN METHODS OF CONTRACEPTION IN THE UK

No Method	19 per cent
Combined Pill	20 per cent
Mini Pill	4 per cent
Progestogen injection	1 per cent
Condom	24 per cent
Diaphragm	2 per cent
Coil	4 per cent
Natural Methods	1 per cent
Male Sterilization	12 per cent
Female Sterilization	8 per cent
Hysterectomy	5 per cent

* Source: The Durex Report 1994.

Previous research showed that 1 in 10 males rely on the female to provide the condoms!

The failure rates of different methods of contraception are detailed on the opposite page. The figures given are numbers of pregnancies per 100 women using the method for one year, so are effectively percentages.

COITUS INTERRUPTUS

Coitus interruptus, also known as the Withdrawal Method, is one of the oldest male methods of contraception. It received a bad press in Biblical days when Onan 'spilled his seed' on the ground rather than fulfil his obligation to impregnate his dead brother's wife. For this defiance of the Torah he was struck down on the spot.

Coitus interruptus involves the male withdrawing his penis from the female just before ejaculation. Withdrawal requires strong motivation as the instinctive male reaction at impend

Method	Failure rates	
	Lowest expected	Typical
No contraception	85	85
Withdrawal	4	18
Female fertility awareness	2	>20
Diaphragm	6	2–15
Spermicides alone	3	21
Sponge	6	9–25
Male condom	2	2–15
Female condom	N/A	12–15
Coil (IUCD)	1	1–3
Progestogen coil	2	N/A
Combined Pill	0.1	1–7
Mini Pill	0.5	1–4
Progestogen injection	<1	<1
Progestogen implant	<1	<1
Female sterilization	0.2	0.4
Male sterilization	0.1	0.15
Morning-after Pill	1–4	1–4
Morning-after IUCD	1	2

ing orgasm is to thrust as far into the female as possible.

Timing is also important. If withdrawal occurs too early, orgasm will fail. If too late, semen will enter the vagina. Even if the timing is right, often some sperm are released early along with the lubricating secretions from Cowper's glands. Withdrawal should not be relied on if it is imperative that pregnancy is avoided.

Having said that, if practised carefully coitus interruptus is surprisingly effective. Some studies have found no difference in failure rates between the withdrawal method and barrier methods such as the diaphragm. Although there are many better methods of contraception available, withdrawal is better than nothing in an emergency situation.

The effectiveness of coitus interruptus is improved with the additional use of spermicides.

THE CONDOM

History

The (male) condom was supposedly invented by the Italian anatomist, Fallopius, in the sixteenth century. He prescribed linen sheaths impregnated with lotion to protect uncircumcised males from the ravages of syphilis. These were fitted over the tip of the penis (glans) and the foreskin was pulled over them. The contraceptive side-effect was only noticed later by accident.

By the eighteenth century, condoms were still used against syphilis, although Casanova donned condoms made from sheep intestines or fish skin '... to put the fair sex under shelter from all fear'.

A mid-nineteenth-century recipe for a condom commanded a man to:

> Take the caecum of a sheep; soak it first in water, turn it on both sides, then repeat the operation in a weak solution of soda, which must be changed every four or five hours, for five or six successive times; then remove the mucous membrane with the nail; sulphur, wash in clean water, and then in soap and water; rinse, inflate and dry. Next cut it to the required length and attach a piece of ribbon to the open end. Use to prevent infection or pregnancy.

Interestingly, five antique condoms recently went up for auction at Christie's. Three painted with erotic scenes from the mid-nineteenth century fetched prices of £2,400 each, and an illustrated French version attracted a record sum of £3,300.

The modern sheath was supposedly invented by a Dr Condom, court physician to King Charles II. It is more likely that the term *condom* derives from the Latin for receptacle – *condus*.

In the 1880s the birth rate in Britain and Europe declined. One suggested reason was the availability of reusable contraceptive prophylactics which were sensually acceptable, relatively unobtrusive and not malodorous, although they did not fit at all well. Their respectability was presumably enhanced by sporting full-colour pictures of Queen Victoria on the packaging.

Modern Condoms

Modern condoms are made from highest quality pre-lubricated latex. Worldwide, there are two standard widths (52 mm and 49 mm) and several different lengths. Non-lubricated condoms are also available, as are condoms lubricated with nonoxynol-9 spermicide, or with a non-spermicidal lubricant (sk-70) for those allergic to spermicides. They can sport ribs and knobbles, feature a variety of colours or flavours and some even glow in the dark. Perhaps the ultimate invention is the musical condom. Designed for the tone-sensitive, it contains a piezo-electric sound transducer microchip and can play any melody or voice message. A US patent has been granted. There is even a condom just invented which plays a tune if it breaks during intercourse!

With careful use, condoms have a 2 per cent failure rate. If roughly handled or not put on as soon as sexual activity is started, failure rates can soar to 15 per cent. Approximately one in 12 male sheaths burst during use, despite electronic testing of integrity. Bursting is more likely during dry sex when a water-based lubricant has not been used. Sheaths are best used with a water-based spermicidal jelly to provide additional protection in the case of condom failure.

Only water-based lubricants (e.g. KY Jelly) are recommended for use with latex condoms. Mineral-based oils (e.g. baby oil, petroleum jelly, some spermicidal creams) weaken latex and may even dissolve it. Tests have shown that mineral oils can reduce condom strength by up to 95 per cent within 15 minutes.

Assessing Condom Reliability

In the UK, quality condoms carry a British Standards Institute Kite Mark BS 3704 (1989) or the stricter European Standard (ISO 4074). A new, stricter British Standard has also just been agreed. Those that glow in the dark ('fundoms'), sport 'go-faster' stripes or are labelled 'not to be used as a barrier' should not be relied upon.

How to Use a Condom

It may seem obvious how to use a condom, but a study involving almost 300 men asked to put a condom on a model penis showed that:

- 16 men had not used condoms before, yet only one of these read the instructions. Overall, only 1.7 per cent bothered to read the instruction leaflet supplied.
- 13 per cent of men were careless when opening the foil wrapper, increasing the risk of tearing the condom.
- 20 per cent of men tried unrolling the condom inside out.
- 3 per cent of men unrolled the condom over their finger and tried pulling it on like a sock.
- Nearly 40 per cent of men did not squeeze the teat. If the teat is not squeezed, air gets trapped in the condom, increasing the risk of semen leakage along the condom.
- Only 50 per cent of the men tested were assessed as having no problem putting the condom on the model.
- 12 per cent of men (mostly aged 16–24) were assessed as having obvious difficulty in using a condom.
- 20 per cent of men who had never used a condom before – or who had not used one within a year – had difficulty applying the condom to the model.

WHAT TO DO

1. Avoid any genital-to-genital contact until the condom covers the penis, as some sperm are released early during sexual activity.
2. Always check the use-by (expiry) date on the packet.
3. Open the foil packet carefully so the condom isn't damaged. Once an airtight wrapping is opened deterioration is rapid, so

don't use a condom whose wrapping is cracked or torn. Ultraviolet light, heat, humidity and ozone can all cause latex to deteriorate.

4. Squeeze the teat of the condom to expel any air.
5. While still squeezing the teat, unroll the condom over the erect penis using your other hand. Don't attempt to apply it if the penis is not fully erect and don't unroll the condom before trying to put it on.
6. Make sure the condom is completely rolled down and extends to the base of the penis. This is important – if not pulled down completely it may ruck up during intercourse and come off.
7. If a lubricant is needed, make sure it is water-based (e.g. KY Jelly).
8. Immediately after ejaculation, grasp the penis and condom near the base and hold firmly while withdrawing the penis.
9. Don't continue penetration until you lose erection as this increases the risk of spilling sperm.
10. Gently slide the condom off, taking care not to spill any sperm. Wrap the used condom in a tissue and dispose of it hygienically. If you tie a knot in it, it will not flush down the toilet very easily.
11. Use each condom only once.

TIPS

- If you are not confident using a condom, try practising alone first.
- Don't put a condom on until the penis is fully erect.
- Don't initiate genital-to-genital contact until the condom is on.
- Always use a spermicidal jelly with condoms. This greatly increases their protection against pregnancy. Nonoxynol-9 also helps to protect against gonorrhoea, Chlamydia (NSU), syphilis, herpes and HIV.
- Only use water-based lubricants.
- Carry several condoms, not just one.
- Use a condom for protection against sexually transmissible diseases, even if contraception is not necessary.

Condom Size

A tightly fitting condom is more likely to burst than one that fits correctly. One study suggested that the British standard condom width of 52 mm measured flat is too small for approximately half of Western penises, who need a flat condom width of 64 mm.

A UK questionnaire of 281 males found that 25 per cent had difficulty putting condoms on, and of these, 19 per cent admitted it was because they were too tight. As a result, 73 per cent had experienced a condom coming off and 68 per cent had experienced condoms splitting on them. There is a strong case for condoms to be manufactured in a wider range of sizes.

A new polyurethane condom that is twice as strong as a latex one as well as being thinner, non-allergenic and which will not dissolve in petroleum jelly is being tested in the US. It should be on general sale in the UK in 1995.

VASECTOMY

Vasectomy is the contraceptive choice for around 15 per cent of sexually active males. Worldwide, 42 million couples rely on this method of contraception; in the UK, around 40,000 vasectomies are performed each year. Of these, it is estimated that around 2% are reversed per year.

Vasectomy can be performed under a local or general anaesthetic. A few operations have been performed using hypnosis or acupuncture for pain control.

In the traditional vasectomy, a midline incision is made in the scrotum – although some surgeons make a small cut on each side. The two vas deferens, one arising from each testicle, are then identified and a small section pulled out through the incision. A small length is clamped and cut and the two cut ends securely tied. Altogether, vasectomy usually takes less than 20 minutes, and is usually completed within 10 minutes.

Several refinements of this technique are used. The cut ends of the vas deferens may be sealed by heat rather than tied.

Other surgeons loop the cut end back on itself and stitch it to prevent spontaneous rejoining of the ends. Yet others slip one cut end behind an anatomical membrane (fascia) so that it cannot come into contact with the other cut end on that side.

The Li vasectomy, perfected in China, is a no-scalpel technique. The vas is gripped through the scrotal skin by a ringed instrument and the overlying scrotum punctured with a sharp pair of dissecting forceps. The vas deferens are individually fished out to be cut and sealed. The small puncture in the scrotal skin is pinched tightly for a minute and then swabbed with anaesthetic. No stitches are required and the procedure is quick, with less risk of complications than with traditional methods.

The newest technique is a non-surgical, easily reversible vasectomy. Under local anaesthetic, the vas deferens are gripped through the scrotal skin by a special clamp. The vas is then injected with a freshly prepared elastomer liquid which hardens over 10–20 minutes. This forms a pliable but non-adherent plug about the size of a grain of rice which blocks the central bore of the vas deferens.

In China, over 12,000 men have had this procedure; a success rate of 98 per cent has been quoted. For easy reversal, a small slit is made over the scrotum under local anaesthetic and the elastomer plug is squeezed out.

After the Vasectomy

Immediately after the operation the man is usually advised to rest for 24 hours and to avoid strenuous activities for a few days. Paracetamol usually controls any discomfort and is better than aspirin, which may prolong bleeding. Most men are able to return to work within 24 hours and to resume an active sex life (using a temporary method of contraception such as the condom) when they feel like it. Tight-fitting underpants or an athletic jockstrap are often advised for use during the first 48 hours (or longer if necessary) to support the scrotum and minimize discomfort.

Early Complications of Vasectomy

Complications of vasectomy are rare but can include bleeding, swelling and bruising (haemotoma). The scrotum may turn blue or black, or may harden and become intensely painful – usually if instructions to rest are not followed. If bleeding continues, an exploratory operation to tie off the bleeding vessel may rarely be needed.

Occasionally, the operative site becomes infected. Swelling, redness, pain and fever depend on the severity of the infection. Any infection needs urgent antibiotics to prevent epididymo-orchitis (*see page 32*).

Vasectomy Lag Period

A vasectomy is not immediately effective as a method of contraception. The vas deferens is a sperm storage duct and it takes at least three months (15–30 ejaculations) to clear out the current 'lodgers'. Semen samples are checked monthly from three months after the operation until three ejaculates have been declared free of sperm. Alternative methods of contraception must be used until the man is told the vasectomy may be relied upon. It is then wise to have a semen analysis once per year.

Failure of Vasectomy

The cut ends of the vas deferens can spontaneously rejoin soon after the operation. This most commonly occurs 10–14 weeks after the operation, although cases of recanalization (as this is known) occurring 12 years later have been reported.

The failure rate of vasectomy is usually quoted as 1 in 2,000. In skilled hands, where the surgeon separates the two cut ends of each vas by placing them either side of a sheet of tissue called the spermatic fascia, the chance of regaining spontaneous fertility (by the two ends coming together and rejoining) is an order of magnitude less, at 1 in 10,000. Nor does this technique affect the chances of successful future reversal.

One case has been cited where a vasectomized man with scanty, occasional motile sperm in his ejaculate (therefore considered infertile) managed to impregnate his wife three years after a vasectomy. DNA and other tests suggested he was 99.999 per cent likely to have been the father.

Vasectomy and Future Health

There is no evidence that having a vasectomy increases the risk of sexual problems, that it changes testosterone hormone levels or decreases sex drive.

Within the last few years, researchers have suggested that vasectomy increased the risk of prostate cancer. After much examination of the data, US health experts declared there was no biological evidence to suggest this. The risk of developing prostate cancer after vasectomy was considered too small to justify any changes in medical practice and it was recommended that doctors should continue to offer and perform vasectomies.

Sixty per cent of vasectomized males do develop antibodies that cause sperm clumping. Testicular biopsies of the testes after vasectomy show that spermatogenesis is disrupted and fibrosis (scarring) of the testes occurs in some cases. Many of these patients were subsequently proved fertile, however, so the importance of these changes is difficult to assess. Sperm granulomas (immunological swellings) below the area where the tubes were tied may cause small, painful lumps in some males, and 1 per cent of men complain of prolonged pain following the operation. This is probably due to distension of the epididymes.

Three studies have suggested a link between vasectomy and future development of testicular cancer. Other studies have found no such association and the risk is not thought to be significant. More studies are needed, however, to evaluate the long-term risks of vasectomy.

Reversal of Vasectomy

A vasectomy should always be assumed permanent when a man first decides to undergo the procedure. In practice, however, 2 per cent of vasectomies are reversed per year due to future, unforeseen changes in circumstance.

The skill of the surgeon and the length of time that has passed since the original vasectomy are the biggest factors in determining a successful outcome.

Reversal of vasectomy is a relatively long procedure, taking 90–120 minutes. It is performed under either local or general anaesthesia. Men who are having a second attempt at reversal, or those with anatomical irregularities (e.g. hernia, varicocoele) usually receive a general anaesthetic.

The cut ends of each vas must be identified and the scarred, tied or burned tissues trimmed. Once the central bore (lumen) of each vas deferens is opened, the epididymis on that side is gently squeezed to check that sperm are siphoning up through. This rules out any blockages further down. The tubes are then flushed with saline to remove debris and the ends painstakingly sewn together. Chances of success are greatest where a specialist uses micro-surgical techniques and magnification (using an operating microscope). The vas channel being rejoined is only 0.25 to 0.33 mm in diameter, and 90 per cent of the thickness of the tube consists of the muscular walls. Often the testicular end of the tube has dilated due to the pressure of semen build-up, and additional skill is required to join the ends of tubes with different bores.

Tiny stitches are inserted to join the inner walls of the two trimmed ends. These must be placed skilfully to oppose the ends exactly and to minimize the formation of scar tissue. Several larger stitches then bring the thick outer walls of the vas together.

Following the original vasectomy, immunological and inflammatory processes can lead to tissue changes within the testes. The build-up and reabsorption of sperm can lead to swellings (sperm granulomas) forming in each epididymis, which may interfere with semen flow once the vasectomy is reversed.

Vasectomy also introduces the risk of a man making auto-antibodies against his own sperm, rendering them sluggish and interfering with future fertility should the vasectomy be reversed.

Different surgeons have different success rates for reversal of vasectomy. These vary from 40 per cent to 90 per cent success in restoring sperm passage through the vas deferens, and a 30 per cent to 50 per cent chance of the man fathering a child. The odds are significantly reduced if the vasectomy was performed more than 10 years previously.

Following a reversal of vasectomy, men often have a lower sperm count than achieved before the original operation. There is an improvement in sperm count, viability and motility over the first year.

If conception does not occur, sperm from the ejaculate (or aspirated from the epididymis) can be harvested and concentrated for use in assisted fertility techniques such as *in vitro* fertilization.

EMERGENCY CONTRACEPTION

All males should be aware of the existence of female methods of emergency (so-called 'morning after') contraception. These may prove necessary when a condom bursts or when the withdrawal method fails.

The morning after pill is more flexible than it sounds and can be started within 72 hours of unprotected sex. The female takes two tablets as soon as possible within 72 hours of the unprotected sex. Two more tablets are then taken 12 hours later. This emergency pill has a 4 per cent failure rate.

In some cases, a woman can also have a contraceptive coil inserted into her womb up to five days following unprotected sex.

10

SEXUALLY TRANSMISSIBLE DISEASES

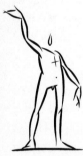 Despite the widespread publicity about HIV and safer sex, sexually transmissible diseases (STDs) remain common. During 1992–93, 327,000 males attended genito-urinary clinics in the UK, a 1 per cent increase on the previous year. This figure does not include the increasingly large number of men who choose to receive treatment for an STD from their doctor rather than at a special genito-urinary clinic.

It is now widely known that sexual activity without a condom while abroad is a high risk activity for catching a number of STDs, including HIV and hepatitis B. Despite this, the attitude that 'It won't happen to me' is common.

A study at a UK genito-urinary clinic found that 51 per cent of heterosexual males had sex with a local foreign contact while on holiday during the preceding year. Many did not use a condom. Study of a further 68 males returning from abroad with an STD found that only 32 per cent had used condoms. Seven per cent said the condom had burst or come off, 12 per cent had not used them consistently, and 49 per cent hadn't bothered with a condom at all.

Nearer to home, a survey of 1,000 young people aged 16 to 29 found that 600 admitted to having sex with a new partner while on holiday in Devon without using a condom.

The sexual behaviour of homosexual males in England and Wales is hardly better. Gonorrhoea, syphilis, HIV and hepatitis B are slowly increasing in incidence, as unsafe sex is just as common now as it was five years ago. In particular, research shows that some HIV-positive men continue to practise unsafe sex despite the fact that they are receiving counselling on living with the virus. This shows a bizarre lack of concern for their own health and that of others.

SAFER SEX

A man's main protection against HIV, hepatitis B and other STDs is practising safer sex. Any sexual activity, even safer sex, with at-risk partners (e.g. bisexuals, drug abusers, casual contacts abroad or with those from endemic countries) greatly increases your risk of contracting HIV or hepatitis B.

- Always use strong, reliable condoms unless in a monogamous relationship where you know your partner is not infected with hepatitis B or HIV.
- Keep your number of sexual partners to a minimum, especially when travelling abroad.
- Avoid activities in which bleeding can occur (e.g. anal sex, fisting).
- Only use water-based lubricants. Oil-based products such as baby oil or petroleum jelly can weaken rubber condoms by 95 per cent within 15 minutes.
- Use condoms and/or dental dams for oral sex.
- Avoid sharing needles, razors, toothbrushes or sex toys such as vibrators.
- If travelling to endemic areas, carry 'dedicated medical kits' (specially put together for people travelling to risk areas) containing syringes and needles, etc. Some travellers take their own transfusion kits and substitute blood products.
- Have a dental and medical check-up before travelling, to

167

minimize the risk of having to be treated abroad.
- Even if both you and your partner are HIV positive, still practise safer sex. Reinfection with HIV, or superinfection with herpes or hepatitis B will cause further harm to your health and may hasten the progress of your disease.

EXOTIC VENEREAL DISEASES THAT CAN BE ACQUIRED ABROAD

Several exotic STDs are occasionally seen in the UK, having been caught in the tropics. These include:

Chancroid
due to infection with the bacterium *Haemophilus ducreyii*. This causes painful genital ulcers within three to five days of infection. The lymph nodes in the groin swell up to cause painful, bulging swellings (nicknamed 'buboes'). In severe cases, extensive tissue ulceration and destruction occur.

Lymphogranuloma venereum
caused by *Chlamydia trachomatis serotypes 1, 2 and 3*, which are closely related to the Chlamydia that causes non-specific urethritis *(see page 77)*. Small, painless ulcers or lumps appear 7–15 days after infection. Fever, headache, muscle and joint aches and a rash sometimes also occur.

   This first stage is short-lived and is occasionally symptomless. The disease then progresses to massive swelling and inflammation of the lymph nodes in the groin to form unilateral or bilateral buboes. Abscesses may form with ulcers on the overlying skin. These take several months to heal unless antibiotic treatment is given.

Granuloma inguinale (Donovanosis)
due to an organism called *Donovania granulomatis*. This causes painless nodules 1–12 weeks after infection. They are commonly sited on the penis or around the anus. The nodules

gradually ulcerate to form painless, beef-red ulcers with a typical rolled edge. Bleeding often occurs as the ulcer slowly enlarges. Antibiotics (e.g. tetracycline) will cure the infection but, if left untreated, ulcers may eventually heal with massive scarring.

CHLAMYDIA AND NON-SPECIFIC URETHRITIS

Infection with Chlamydia trachomatis is the commonest male STD in the Western world. It causes up to 60 per cent of cases of non-specific urethritis (NSU) and 45 per cent of cases of epididymo-orchitis (*see page 32*). It can also be isolated from 7 per cent of sexually active males attending genito-urinary clinics who do not have symptoms of infection.

In the UK 43,294 males were diagnosed as having NSU during 1992–93. A further 12,806 cases were definitely attributed to Chlamydia and a further 3,629 men were treated for the condition 'epidemiologically' because their partners were affected. This was despite their having no symptoms themselves.

Chlamydia is a cross between a bacterium and a virus. It is too small to be seen under a light microscope and is difficult to grow in culture. Most clinics detect it with a special antigen test performed on sloughed urethral lining cells – a test that can take several days to give a result.

Some men infected with Chlamydia have no symptoms but can pass on the infection to female (or male) sexual partners. Other men notice symptoms of stinging at the end of the penis, watery discharge and pain on passing water. These symptoms usually start within one to six weeks of exposure to infection.

Infected males often complain of a discharge early in the morning which clears during the day. Staining of the under-clothes with a mucous or slightly pus-stained discharge is another give-away sign. Sometimes, urination produces a spray as the end of the gummed-up urethra bursts open as water is forced through.

A tentative diagnosis is made by taking a swab of the

urethral discharge and examining it under the microscope. Pus cells are usually found but no causative bacteria. Diagnosis is also helped by collecting urine in three specimen jars. Haziness of the first urine passed which doesn't clear on adding 5 per cent acetic acid (vinegar) indicates there are pus cells suspended in it. Threads of pus and sloughed urethral lining cells can often be fished out too and examined under the microscope. Urethral swabs are also sent off for antigen testing. Urethral lining cells are needed, and these are obtained by passing a small plastic ringed probe 2 cm down into the urethra and gently twisting it around. This is unpleasant, especially if the urethra is inflamed.

The presence of pus cells in a urethral discharge but no causative organisms merits a diagnosis of non-specific urethritis (NSU), which is likely to be due to Chlamydia.

Treatment is started immediately with a course of antibiotics (one of the many types of tetracycline or erythromycin) while awaiting results of the antigen tests. These can take several days to arrive and do not always find traces of infection when it is there. It is better to treat a suspected but unproved Chlamydia infection, than to let a missed infection grumble on.

If left untreated, Chlamydia can progress to epididymo-orchitis (infection and swelling of a testicle) or can spread to the eye (usually by the fingers) to cause conjunctivitis. NSU also triggers an immunological reaction called Reiter's syndrome in 1 per cent of affected males.

Reiter's Syndrome

Reiter's syndrome is diagnosed by the presence of urethritis, bilateral conjunctivitis (and sometimes uveitis – inflammation of the lining of the eye, including the iris) plus arthritis. Most patients with Reiter's syndrome have a recent history of a new sexual contact followed by urethral inflammation and discharge.

Reiter's syndrome is the commonest cause of arthritis in young men. The arthritis usually affects one or two joints –

commonly a knee or ankle – and is often accompanied by a fever and feelings of being unwell. The affected joints become hot, swollen, stiff and painful. Tendons, ligaments and the soles of the feet may become inflamed. Skin rashes are also common.

Treatment of Reiter's arthritis is with painkillers and anti-inflammatory drugs. The NSU is treated with antibiotics. Most first attacks resolve within two to six months, but recovery can be delayed for as long as a year. Unfortunately, the arthritis flares up again in a third of cases, especially after further episodes of NSU. During 1992–93, a total of 293 males were newly diagnosed as having Reiter's syndrome in the UK.

Chlamydia and Subfertility

Other important reasons for diagnosing and treating Chlamydia infection in males is to trace and treat female contacts and prevent the disease being passed on any further. Chlamydia infection in females is often symptomless and slowly inflames and blocks the Fallopian tubes. This is a common cause of pelvic inflammatory disease (PID) and subsequent female infertility.

Low-grade infection with organisms causing NSU, including Chlamydia, can also trigger male subfertility. This is because pus cells affect the sperm. Increased numbers of superoxide free radicals, which have been linked with sperm damage, are released. This effect is reversible after antibiotic therapy.

It is important not to indulge in sexual activity until treatment has finished and all your tests are clear, otherwise infection can be passed on and can flare up again in yourself.

Other causes of NSU apart from Chlamydia include organisms that are difficult to see or culture such as Ureaplasma and Mycoplasma. These respond to the same antibiotics as Chlamydia. Mycoplasma genitalium was first isolated from two men with NSU 10 years ago but has only recently been confirmed as a causative agent. Using DNA probes, it has recently been identified in 23 per cent of men with symptoms

171

of NSU in whom Chlamydia was not found. Mycoplasma genitalium was also found in 3 per cent of men who had no symptoms of infection.

GENITAL WARTS

Genital warts are one of the commonest STDs to affect males, with infection almost classifiable as an epidemic. During 1992–93, over 49,000 cases were treated among UK males, of which almost 27,000 were first attacks. The other 22,000 cases were recurrent infections.

Genital warts are caused by the human papilloma virus (HPV), of which at least 60 different types exist. Essentially, a wart is a benign tumour. These vary in shape and size from small, multiple, finger-like projections to single, large excrescences that resemble cauliflowers. They are often moist and can itch.

Genital warts are usually transmitted by sexual contact, although it is thought that occasionally the virus is passed on via the hands. After exposure to infection it takes between a few weeks and several years before the first wart suddenly appears. They can occur anywhere on the penis, within the tip of the urethra or around the anus.

HPV can also enter a dormant stage within human cells and, once infection is present, may reoccur periodically throughout life. Some types of HPV are also linked with an increased risk of developing genital cancers. For this reason, women who have had genital warts should have annual cervical smears. In the same way, some experts suggest that homosexual men with anogenital warts should have regular anal canal smears to pick up early cell changes that might eventually lead to anal carcinoma.

Genital warts are best treated in a specialist genito-urinary clinic where you can be screened for evidence of other STDs. Never be too embarrassed to see your doctor about genital warts.

Treatment options include:

- painting the warts with a solution of podophyllum. This is a cytotoxic substance which literally kills wart-infected cells. It is applied to the warts at the clinic and subsequently washed off after six to eight hours. Application is repeated at weekly intervals and can take weeks to remove visible signs of wart infection.
- applying podophyllotoxin, the active ingredient of podophyllum. This can be prescribed in a weak solution for self-application. The solution is painted on twice daily for three days per week over a maximum of five weeks. Again, it takes several weeks to work.
- applying trichloro-acetic acid (TCA) in the clinic on a weekly basis. This strong acid coagulates wart cells and usually works quite quickly. If not applied carefully, ulceration of surrounding skin can occur. TCA and podophyllum are sometimes used together for faster results.
- freezing the warts with a cryotherapy probe. This is best reserved for single warts and those just inside the tip of the urethra, as it is less likely than other methods to cause urethral scarring. Regular repeat sessions are usually needed before the warts disappear.
- burning off the warts using bipolar electrocautery (e.g. ValleyLab). The warts are numbed with a local anaesthetic injection (using a fine dental needle) and then literally exterminated by grasping them between a pair of forceps and passing a buzz of electricity through. Shallow burns form, which heal over the following week to produce instant and gratifying results. This is an excellent method for treating larger or multiple genital warts. Unfortunately, the equipment is expensive and not every genitourinary clinic can afford it.

GENITAL HERPES

Genital herpes was originally thought to be caused only by the *Herpes simplex virus type 2* (HSV2), while cold sores on the lip were thought more likely to be due to Herpes simplex type 1. This distinction has become blurred, however, with the increased practice of oral sex.

Blood tests show that most of us have been exposed to the Herpes simplex virus by the time we reach middle age. Many people have what is called a sub-clinical attack – with no visible signs of infection and no ill affects. These people are then naturally immune to further infection but do not know they have been infected.

In Europe and the US, genital Herpes simplex virus infection is the commonest cause of genital ulceration, accounting for 5 per cent of patients seen in genito-urinary clinics. The US Center for Disease Control estimates that up to 500,000 new cases of genital herpes occur in the US per year. A population survey suggested that the disease may be present in up to 25 million people.

In the UK, the number of genital herpes cases increased by 70 per cent from 1981 to 1985. Between 1992 and 1993, 11,609 males were treated for genital herpes infection, of which 54 per cent were first, or primary, attacks.

Primary Herpes

The first time you catch herpes is known as the *primary attack*. If infection causes symptoms they usually develop two to 14 days after exposure. Symptoms of primary herpes include:

- itching and irritation around the genitals
- a general feeling of being unwell
- low-grade fever
- headache
- muscle aches and joint pains
- abdominal pain
- shooting pains in the lower limbs (neuralgia)
- enlarged, tender lymph nodes (glands) in the groin
- difficulty passing urine.

After one or two days, the classic herpes blister appears as a red, inflamed lump. This quickly breaks down to form a blister which ruptures to leave a painful ulcer.

These lesions are highly infectious and weep fluid that is teeming with over 1,000,000 viruses per ml.

In the male, symptoms usually last for 10–13 days. There is a wide range of clinical patterns, however, and the primary attack may be mild (lasting only a few days) or severe (symptoms lasting three to four weeks). Complete healing usually occurs in under 21 days unless the immune system is compromised in any way.

Ulcers on the glans penis and foreskin of uncircumcised males tend to heal without scars. Lesions in dry areas (e.g. penile shaft, scrotum, thighs, buttocks) crust over and form a scab. These tend to leave faint marks which will fade with time.

Peri-anal and rectal lesions are usually accompanied by spasm of the anus (tenesmus) and a profuse rectal mucous discharge.

Very occasionally it proves impossible to pass water during a primary herpetic attack. The bladder fills up and acute retention of urine occurs. This may be an involuntary reflex due to the pain of hot, acid, salty urine contacting ulcers at the tip of the penis or in the urethral entrance. Relief may be gained by sitting in a warm bath and urinating directly into the bathwater. Sometimes, a local anaesthetic and catheterization is necessary.

The herpes virus can also cause acute urinary retention through temporarily interfering with nerve function as it invades nerve endings. This is known as lumbo-sacral radiculo-myelopathy. In males, it is most common where herpes infection of the rectum and anus (proctitis) is present. Symptoms usually include impotence as well as difficulty urinating and opening the bowels. Catheterization and hospitalization are usually necessary, as symptoms take a week or two to resolve.

Recurrent Genital Herpes

Herpes viruses are unusual in that they are not totally eradicated from the body by the immune system. During the primary attack, the virus enters sensory nerve endings near the site of infection and travel up the associated nerves. They remain dormant within the dorsal root ganglion of the sacral nerves at the base of the spinal cord, out of reach of antibodies or antiviral drugs, until reactivated.

Several factors are known to trigger a herpes recurrence. These include:

- physical stress
- mental stress
- excessive heat or cold
- local genital trauma (e.g. rough sexual intercourse, plucking or shaving pubic hair)
- fluctuations in pituitary and adrenal hormone levels
- general ill health, other infections (e.g. colds)
- impaired immunity (e.g. due to drugs, HIV, cancer)
- exposure to ultra-violet light (e.g. sunbathing)
- exposure to X-irradiation

Upon reactivation, herpes viruses travel down the nerve to reach the genital mucosa. It may not take the same route as the way it came up, which is why a primary attack may consist of lesions on the penis while a recurrence may affect the anal region.

Recurrences are never as bad as the primary attack. You will not get the flu-like symptoms and, often, only a tiny sore appears. This is more of a nuisance than a problem. The sores tend to heal quickly compared with those of the primary attack and are often gone within three to five days.

Frequency of Recurrences

It is impossible to predict how many herpes recurrences someone will suffer. Around 50 per cent of sufferers never have a recurrence, 25 per cent get one once or twice per year, while a few unlucky people seem to get one every month. In general, Herpes simplex recurrences become less frequent with time – infections are said to 'burn themselves out'.

Fifty per cent of patients notice prodromal symptoms (early

warning signs of an impending attack) before recurrent lesions occur. These include itching, tingling, pins and needles, numbness, burning and shooting pains in the buttocks, thighs, penis, scrotum or even the feet. These prodromal symptoms are due to irritation as the Herpes simplex virus travels up or down the sensory nerve axons.

To help prevent triggering a recurrence, avoid strong sunlight or sun beds. Wear loose underwear (e.g. boxer shorts) so air can circulate and keep your genitals cool. Keep a record of when you get recurrent attacks in an attempt to find a pattern. If, for example, recurrences always come when you are over-worked and stressed, try to avoid this. If they are related to rough sex, try using a lubricant such as KY Jelly.

Asymptomatic Shedding

Some people seem to shed the herpes virus without any symptoms. Infectious viral particles have been isolated from the urethra and semen of men who have never even had a primary attack. Some experts now advise people who know they have had genital herpes to use a barrier method of contraception (male condom, female condom, diaphragm) whenever they make love, even when lesions are not present, so that asymptomatic shedding of the virus does not pass infection on.

When lesions are present, sex is best avoided from the start of the prodrome until lesions are fully healed. Condoms that cover the ulcerated area will provide some protection but cannot guarantee that the virus will not be transmitted.

Similarly, oro-genital contact should be avoided whenever lip or genital sores are present. Oral herpes can be passed to the genitals and vice versa.

Treatment of Genital Herpes

During a primary attack of herpes, try to attend a genito-urinary clinic straightaway. A drug called acyclovir is available

177

which, if taken early enough, can shorten your attack and may possibly prevent a recurrence. Unfortunately, the diagnosis is not usually made until lesions are present. By then, the herpes virus has already started to invade nerve endings.

Acyclovir is available as a cream or tablet. It must be used five times per day from the beginning of symptoms, for at least five days.

Take paracetamol or other analgesics to dampen pain, but make sure you keep within the recommended safe doses. If pain is severe, try applying an ice-pack to the sores. Wrap ice cubes in a piece of clean cotton and place on the area for a short while. Use a clean cloth each time – and if possible, wear rubber gloves. Hygiene is important to stop you passing the infection to other parts of your body such as your eyes.

Try bathing the affected area at least four times per day with a salt solution. Make this up by dissolving a tablespoon of salt in a pint of tepid water. Apply the solution for 5–10 minutes, then pat the area dry. A hairdryer set on a low heat can also be used. Leave the sores exposed to air as much as possible, as this avoids irritation from clothes and helps the sores to dry out. If your symptoms are very distressing, your doctor or a genito-urinary clinic can prescribe stronger painkillers.

If recurrent attacks are troublesome, suppression therapy is available. This entails taking continuous acyclovir tablets two to four times a day. Treatment is usually given for three to six months initially to assess the patient's response. On stopping, if a recurrence occurs treatment can begin again.

GONORRHOEA

Gonorrhoea is a sexually transmissible disease caused by the bacterium *Neisseria gonorrhoea*. In the UK, around 8,000 men contract gonorrhoea every year. The number of cases is falling, but a recent increase in rectal gonorrhoea among homosexuals is worrying as it implies a laxer attitude towards safer sex.

The risk of a man catching gonorrhoea following a single episode of unprotected vaginal intercourse with an infected woman is around 20 per cent. This rises to 80 per cent after four exposures. In contrast, a woman is 90 per cent likely to catch it from an infected man following a single episode of sexual activity.

Sexually acquired gonorrhoea can infect the male genito-urinary tract, rectum or throat. A sore throat occurs in 3–7 per cent of heterosexual males and is accompanied by a fever and swollen lymph nodes (glands) in the neck. The rectum is the only site of infection in 40 per cent of cases among male homosexuals. Infection is then asymptomatic in 90 per cent of cases. Only 10 per cent of males seem to develop a mucous-and-blood-stained discharge, itching or pain on opening their bowels.

The usual incubation period for gonorrhoea is two to five days, but sometimes infection remains asymptomatic. The bacteria stick to the outside of cells lining the urethra or other mucous membrane and, within 24 hours, penetrate inside the cell where they start to reproduce.

The usual signs of infection are a heavily pus-stained discharge from the penis and pain on passing water. This pain is commonly described as like peeing broken glass or razor blades. Symptoms seem to have altered within the West over recent years, with gonorrhoea now producing a milder discharge and less pain on passing water. Because of this, it is important to have even mild, transient symptoms checked out as early as possible.

Diagnosis is made by taking swabs of the discharge and examining them microscopically. Staining techniques reveal pus cells with groups of paired bacteria within. The bacteria are quite small and are easily missed. Additional swabs are therefore sent off for culture and to confirm infection.

Once diagnosed, gonorrhoea is treated with a single dose of antibiotics such as ciprofloxacin, ofloxacin or azithromycin. Penicillin-combination drugs given as intramuscular injections or courses of tablets are more traditional alternatives. Some cases of gonorrhoea are resistant to penicillin treatment, especially cases contracted in the Far East and Africa. Because of the possibility of inadequate response to treatment, all sexual activity should be refrained from until three sets of swabs, taken at weekly intervals, are subsequently reported negative.

Undiagnosed gonorrhoea can cause complications of prostatitis *(see page 89)* and epididymo-orchitis *(see page 32)* in up to 10 per cent of males. Chronic infection of the male genital tract can also lead to scarring and difficulty in passing water.

In 1 per cent of infected males, gonococcal bacteria spread throughout the body to cause a skin rash, gonococcal tendinitis and arthritis. Fever, shivering, loss of appetite and joint pains can occur, with severe pain on moving. The infection seems to flit from joint to joint initially, but if allowed to progress pus can build up and joint damage occurs.

Even more rarely, gonococci multiply within the bloodstream to cause septicaemia. This can lead to infection of the brain or heart valves, shock, and even death.

SYPHILIS

At present, syphilis is relatively uncommon. Around 800 males contracted the disease within the UK during 1992–93, mostly as a result of homosexual activity. The incidence of heterosexually acquired syphilis is expected to soar, however. Cases have increased 20–30 fold in parts of the US over the last five years, mainly in the inner cities, and a similar trend is likely in the UK.

Syphilis is a sexually transmissible disease caused by a spiral-shaped bacterium, *Treponema pallidum*. Within hours of infection the motile bacteria have entered the bloodstream and spread all over the body. Nine to 90 days later (usually an average of 21 days) a painless, shallow ulcer develops at the site of infection (this may be on the genitals, finger or tongue). The ulcer has sharply demarcated clean edges and a rubbery feel. It is highly infectious and is known as the primary sore, or chancre. It heals over the next one to two months, and leaves a scar.

After a further six to eight weeks, some people develop a mild flu-like illness and a dusky-pink skin rash. This may involve the palms of the hands and soles of the feet, and is usually accompanied by widespread swollen lymph nodes (glands) and ulceration of mucous membranes (e.g. in the mouth, genitals, anus). The hair may fall out in clumps, and large, flat wart-like growths may appear on the genitals. This secondary stage of the disease is highly infectious, even in patients who do not develop obvious symptoms.

If left untreated, symptoms improve and the disease becomes latent. The infected person is then no longer infectious. Between three and 20 years later, however, the next stage of tertiary syphilis develops. Tissue destruction occurs at various sites, with the production of lesions known as gummas. Classically, the bones, nose, tongue and other parts of the body get eaten away as if 'riddled with worms'. Thankfully, the discovery of antibiotics and diagnostic blood tests makes this end point rare in the Western world. Tertiary syphilis can cause heart complications or produce a form of madness from progressive brain damage and paralysis.

Syphilis is usually diagnosed and treated once the first chancre appears. Penicillin is the antibiotic of choice and is given as an intramuscular injection daily for around 12 days in the primary stage or for 15 days for treating secondary or latent infection. There is no evidence of resistance to treatment.

Half the people treated with penicillin suffer a reaction within 6–12 hours of the first injection due to the poisons released by the large number of Treponema bacteria killed. This reaction is usually mild (headache, fever, malaise) but is occasionally severe.

HEPATITIS B

Hepatitis B is well known as a disease that is transmitted via contaminated blood. It is also known as a disease that is sexually transmissible during certain homosexual activities. What is less widely appreciated, however, is that hepatitis B is now one of the major STDs among heterosexual males. It is highly infectious and, for patients who survive the acute attack, there is the possibility of long-term serious consequences such as cirrhosis, liver failure and even hepatic (liver) cancer.

Worldwide, the World Health Organization estimates that 2,000 million (2 billion) people are infected with the hepatitis B virus (HBV) – while those infected with HIV is several orders of magnitude less, at 10–12 million.

In the US, around 75,000 cases of heterosexually acquired hepatitis B occur every year. In the UK, this figure is closer to 500 cases per year.

HBV is transmitted in a similar manner to HIV. It is 100 times more infectious than HIV, is transmitted 8.6 times more efficiently and kills more people. It causes an acute inflammation of the liver with jaundice and severe systemic illness. One per cent of patients with acute hepatitis B infection die from overwhelming liver failure. Of those that survive, 10 per cent remain highly infectious, with viral particles present in their blood, semen and saliva. These carriers are the source of other sexually-acquired infections.

Of chronic HBV carriers, up to 50 per cent eventually develop cirrhosis of the liver and they are also 400 times more likely to develop liver cancer than uninfected males. Half of all carriers will eventually die from the long-term complications of their illness.

HBV and its effects are the ninth most common cause of death worldwide, with 2 million people dying each year. Disease surveillance studies in the US have found that approximately 35 per cent of patients with HBV are infected by their sexual partners. Since 1985, the number of cases of HBV in homosexual males has dramatically reduced by over 60 per cent. In contrast, the number of cases of hepatitis B in heterosexuals has increased by 38 per cent, and heterosexual activity now accounts for at least 25 per cent of new cases.

In studies in which heterosexual partners of patients with acute hepatitis B are followed for up to 12 months, the risk of catching the disease through normal heterosexual intercourse is quoted as between 20 and 42 per cent.

The risk of catching HBV is related to the number of sexual partners, duration of sexual activity and personal history of other STDs. Men who have had more than 10 sexual partners throughout their lives have a sixfold risk of catching HBV compared with men who have had two or fewer partners.

HBV is more prevalent abroad than in the UK. In parts of Africa, Asia and the Pacific, 20 per cent of the local population are infectious carriers of HBV. Sex while abroad – especially unprotected sex – is a high risk activity for HBV as well as HIV.

HBV is a frightening disease yet, unlike HIV, it is largely avoidable through vaccination. If you are at risk of coming into contact with blood through your occupation, your employer is obliged to inform you about the risks and to offer vaccination. You are well advised to take the offer up. Vaccinations against HBV are safe. The most modern form is genetically engineered and produced by yeast cells – it is not a blood-derived product.

If you are at risk of HBV through sexual activity (heterosexual or homosexual) it is also worth having vaccination to protect yourself from this dreadful disease. This is not an alternative to practising safer sex, but a safety net to increase your level of protection.

Vaccination Against HBV

- The standard course anti-HBV immunization takes six months. One injection is given straightaway, a second injection one month later and a third injection six months after the first. Adequate immunity may not develop for a further six months after the course is completed.
- An accelerated HBV vaccination schedule is available for travellers. The third dose is given two months after the first and a fourth, booster dose given 12 months later.
- For post-exposure prophylaxis, specific HBV immunoglobulin can be given along with an HBV vaccination within 48 hours of exposure to infection.
- Always have a blood test six months to a year after the course of injections to make sure it has 'taken'. The rate of protection is 90–95 per cent in healthy young adults, but males, the elderly and the overweight may need further booster shots.

183

SEXUAL BEHAVIOUR RISKS FOR HBV

High risk:

- anal or vaginal intercourse without a condom
- oral contact with semen (fellatio with ejaculation)
- sharing sex toys without a condom
- any activity that exposes you to contaminated blood, such as sharing toothbrushes, razors, needles; unscreened blood transfusions; dental or medical interventions abroad.

Medium to high risk:

- anal or vaginal intercourse with a condom
- fellatio without ejaculation
- wet kissing (e.g. intimate mouth-to-mouth)

Lower risk:
- mutual masturbation

Minimal Risk:
- dry kissing (e.g. mouth-to-cheek)

HIV AND AIDS

The Acquired Immune Deficiency Syndrome (AIDS) is caused by infection with the Human Immunodeficiency Virus (HIV). This invades a type of white blood cell known as a CD4 (helper) lymphocyte and damps down the body's immune response to infection and rogue cancer cells.

There are two different types of HIV: HIV-1 and HIV-2. Some people are infected with both viruses. As the virus can mutate readily, different strains of HIV-1 and HIV-2 are constantly being identified.

Worldwide, at least 13 million people are HIV positive. The largest number of cases occur in sub-Saharan Africa (over 8 million).

In the US, at least a million people are HIV positive; in New York City AIDS is the commonest cause of death in young males. AIDS first appeared in the UK in 1982 and around 4,000 new cases of male HIV infection are diagnosed every year. There may be 10 times this number who remain undiagnosed and unaware of their status. Seventy per cent of the known cases are in the London area. The Department of Health estimates that, by 1997, HIV- and AIDS-related illnesses will be the third most significant cause of death in the UK in people under 65.

The World Health Organization predict that 40 million people will have been infected with HIV by the year 2000. Worldwide, it is estimated that one new case of infection occurs every 15–20 seconds, and that an AIDS victim dies every 12 minutes.

The Symptoms of HIV infection

The initial stages of infection with HIV are asymptomatic. After two to three months, the body mounts a weak antibody attack against the virus but, in most cases, this is not enough to clear infection. These antibodies are a useful sign that a person has been exposed to HIV infection, however, and can be detected through blood (or saliva) testing. If antibodies are present in the blood, a person is said to be HIV (antibody) positive. The appearance of HIV antibodies in the blood of someone who was previously HIV-negative is known as sero-conversion.

Some people develop a non-specific, short-lived illness similar to glandular fever (mononucleosis) as the body sero-converts. This acute illness occurs two to six weeks after infection and consists of fever, sore throat, lethargy and joint pain. Glands (lymph nodes) may be enlarged. Sometimes a non-specific viral rash also occurs on the trunk and upper limbs. This illness is usually dismissed as a community virus ('just something that is going around') and only a high index of suspicion will lead to early diagnosis. For some reason, this early stage is more commonly reported in Australia than in the

UK or US.

Some people who are HIV positive remain symptom-free for many years. Others develop vague symptoms such as weight loss, fever, night sweats or unexplained diarrhoea. This is known as AIDS-related complex (ARC).

As HIV becomes increasingly active, it invades and kills increasing numbers of the immune CD4 cells. The number of CD4 cells drop and, eventually, the ability to fight infection is impaired. Sufferers can then no longer fight off infections and become prey to a number of exotic illnesses which do not normally trouble healthy humans. This state is known as full-blown AIDS.

Symptoms that suggest AIDS has developed include recurrent infections (e.g. oral thrush, skin fungi, persistent herpes, atypical pneumonias), hairy leukoplakia (white, hairy-looking plaques on the tongue or inner cheek) and Kaposi's sarcoma – a purplish-red form of cancer that forms lesions on the skin or internal organs.

New research suggests that a sizable number of HIV-infected males will experience very little disease progression for many years. Out of 562 men in San Francisco, 31 per cent had not developed AIDS after 10 years of infection and 12 per cent still had normal CD4 counts.

In Milan, a study of 111 infected males led researchers to estimate that 20 per cent would remain symptom free 25 years after initial infection with HIV. Research is ongoing to identify factors in the immune system or lifestyle that might help to prevent the disease's progression.

Transmission of HIV

HIV has been isolated from blood, saliva, breast milk, vaginal secretions and semen. It can be spread in the following ways:

- through infected blood, via:
  - sharing dirty needles; sharing razors
  - blood transfusions in countries where blood is not screened for

HIV, and where sterile equipment is not used
  • dental treatment where equipment is not adequately sterilized
• from an infected mother to her child, either during the birth or through breast feeding.
• through sexual transmission, where an infected partner (male or female) has unprotected intercourse (gay or straight).

Sexual Transmission of HIV

The World Health Organization estimates that 80–90 per cent of people who are HIV positive have contracted the virus through heterosexual sex. It seems that the virus is more easily transmitted from a man to a woman than vice versa. Studies show that around 32 per cent of an infected man's heterosexual partners contract the virus, compared with 25 per cent of an infected woman's male partners.

During fellatio, those who swallow semen are at high risk of HIV infection. The risk of catching HIV via saliva alone is probably small – but significant.

Any bleeding from the gums or vagina (e.g. sores, menstruation) during sexual activity is a high risk factor for transmission of HIV (and hepatitis B infection if present).

Some experts now recommend that oral sex should be avoided unless you definitely know your partner is HIV (and hepatitis B) negative. If you do indulge, condoms or dental dams (bubble-gum flavoured latex squares placed over the female genitalia) provide some protection.

Barrier methods of contraception (male condom, female condom) can protect against HIV during normal sexual activity, and should be used whenever possible. Men who practise anal sex should use extra strong condoms. The spermicide non-oxynol-9 also has some useful anti-HIV properties.

Part Two

ILLNESS AND DISEASE

11

CORONARY HEART DISEASE

Coronary heart disease (CHD) is one of the biggest killers in the Western world, accounting for at least a third, if not half, of all male deaths.

CHD results from the hardening and furring up of the coronary artery walls. This reduces blood flow and leads to less oxygen reaching the heart tissues. In the case of heart muscle, which beats over 100,000 times per day, lack of oxygen rapidly leads to muscle cramping. This causes a characteristic tight, crushing pain known as angina. If the lack of oxygen is extreme, muscle cells will die and a heart attack occurs.

SUDDEN CHEST PAIN

Sudden chest pain should always be taken seriously and medical assistance sought without delay. If it is due to a heart attack, the first two hours are critical. If treatment can restore the blood supply to the damaged muscle by opening up a blocked coronary artery, the tissue can be saved. The classic characteristics of a heart attack include:

- sudden, severe, central chest pain which feels crushing, like being caught in a vice
- pain that often begins at rest (e.g. while you are sitting down) and gets worse on exertion – but it can occur at any time
- pain that may spread up into the jaw or down the arms, usually on the left-hand side
- Breathlessness, pallor and sweating, and a sensation of impending doom. You may also feel an overwhelming need to open your bowels.

When classic symptoms are present the diagnosis is straightforward. But sometimes, especially in the elderly, a heart attack may just cause sudden tiredness, an irregular pulse or heart pump failure with breathlessness and swollen ankles.

RISK FACTORS FOR CHD

Coronary heart disease is linked with several risk factors. The most significant are:

- being male
- having a family history of heart disease
- smoking cigarettes
- having uncontrolled high blood pressure
- eating a diet high in saturated fat
- being obese
- having a high blood LDL-cholesterol
- following a sedentary lifestyle with little exercise
- having poorly controlled diabetes.

A recent survey in the UK found that seven out of every eight adult men show CHD risk factors. Half the adult male population is overweight, with 12 per cent classified as obese. One in six has high blood pressure, one in five has taken no exercise during the preceding four weeks and seven out of 10 have a harmfully raised blood cholesterol level. The survey also showed that men aged 55–74 were more than twice as likely to have suffered a heart attack or stroke than a woman of the same age.

Only 12 per cent of men in the survey were free of the four major risk factors – smoking, high blood pressure, raised cholesterol and lack of exercise.

Other studies show that one in every 10,000 apparently healthy adult males dies suddenly each year in the UK. In 95 per cent of cases this is due to an unexpected heart attack or abnormal heart rhythm triggered by CHD.

CHOLESTEROL AND CHD

Cholesterol is a type of fat unique to the animal kingdom. It is essential for healthy cell membranes, nerve conduction, water-resistant skin and the rapid healing of wounds. Cholesterol is also a vital building block in the manufacture of bile acids and steroid hormones such as testosterone.

Most of our blood cholesterol is synthesized by our liver from saturated fats in our diet. Preformed dietary cholesterol makes only a small contribution to total blood cholesterol levels.

Cholesterol travels around the body in the bloodstream where it is made soluble by joining onto a protein carrier (lipoprotein). It exists in two main forms, high density HDL-cholesterol and low density LDL-cholesterol.

Excessive amounts of LDL-cholesterol are harmful. These molecules are small enough to seep into artery walls and fur them up in a process known as atherosclerosis. Swellings called *plaques* occur which encourage the formation of blood clots. As these grow larger they block small arteries or break off and travel round the bloodstream. Both events are serious and can result in angina, heart attacks, strokes and even death.

HDL-cholesterol, on the other hand, is beneficial. It is too large to pass into artery walls and stays in the bloodstream to transport fats around the body and to neutralize the harmful effects of LDL-cholesterol.

If you are told you have a high blood cholesterol, you need to know how much is in the form of HDL and how much is LDL.

193

If, for example, most of your raised cholesterol is in the form of HDL-cholesterol, you would actually be protected against heart disease.

If your level of LDL-cholesterol is raised, however, you are at increased risk of CHD and must cut back on the amount of saturated fats in your diet. Research suggests that lowering the average blood LDL-cholesterol level by only 10 per cent would prevent a quarter of the CHD deaths occurring in the Western world each year.

Ideally, all males should have their blood cholesterol level checked before the age of 30 and regularly every couple of years thereafter. This is especially important for men who smoke, are overweight, or who have high blood pressure, diabetes or a personal or family history of chest pains, heart attack or hyper-lipidaemia (high fat levels in the blood).

CLASSIFICATION OF TOTAL BLOOD CHOLESTEROL LEVELS

Desirable	< 5.2 mmol/l
Borderline	5.2–6.4 mmol/l
Abnormal	6.5–7.8 mmol/l
High	> 7.8 mmol/l

If total blood cholesterol is abnormal or high, the level will be further analysed to find out how much is in the form of beneficial HDL-cholesterol and how much is harmful LDL-cholesterol.

NORMAL RANGE FOR VARIOUS BLOOD LIPIDS

Total cholesterol	< 5.2 mmol/l
LDL-cholesterol	< 3.5 mmol/l
HDL-cholesterol	> 1 mmol/l
Triglycerides	< 2.3 mmol/l

Slightly stricter criteria apply to men under the age of 30 and for all patients with CHD.

The Treatment of High Blood Cholesterol Levels

Coronary artery disease can be reversed without recourse to drugs or surgery. Diet and lifestyle changes alone can lower cholesterol levels, declog the arteries and help to shrink the atherosclerotic plaques that trigger blood clotting. This was recently shown in 41 patients in California. One group of patients met twice per week for exercise, stress counselling, yoga and meditation. They were advised to follow a vegetarian diet and to get less than 10 per cent of their calories in the form of dietary fat.

The fats they did eat were polyunsaturated and their diet was virtually cholesterol free.

After four years, coronary artery disease was reversed in 72 per cent of patients, with coronary artery narrowing falling from 43.6 to 39.7 per cent.

In contrast, the group that continued with conventional medical advice (to lower fat intake to 30 per cent of calories, obtain less than 200 mg cholesterol in the diet per day, take regular exercise, stop smoking) experienced a worsening of CHD in 87 per cent of patients, with coronary artery narrowing rising from 41.6 to 51.4 per cent.

The improvements were not attributable just to the fall in blood cholesterol levels observed, as these dropped in both groups.

These results are similar to the success achieved by men following a Mediterranean-style diet, who have a 75 per cent lower risk of heart attack.

Beneficial Components of the Mediterranean Diet

The Mediterranean diet is thought to reduce the risk of CHD because it contains olive oil, antioxidant vitamins, garlic, oily fish and red wine, and is high in fibre.

OLIVE OIL

Olive oil (and rapeseed oil) contain vitamin E and are rich in the monounsaturated fat known as oleic acid. This is processed in the body to lower harmful low-density LDL-cholesterol without modifying the desirable high-density HDL-cholesterol. As a result, those who use olive or rapeseed oil regularly (e.g. those of Mediterranean birth or descent) have a lower incidence of CHD.

ANTIOXIDANTS

LDL-cholesterol that has been oxidized by free radical attack is more likely to be absorbed into artery walls and fur them up. By protecting cholesterol against oxidation, antioxidants can protect against CHD.

Research involving 6,000 middle-aged men showed that the risk of developing angina heart pain was three times lower in men with high blood levels of vitamins E, C and betacarotene. Those taking vitamin E supplements had a 12 per cent reduction in CHD. In those who had taken vitamin E for more than two years, their risk of CHD was further reduced by a total of 25 per cent.

A 10-year study in California has shown that a high intake of vitamin C (including the use of supplements) lowers the risk of heart disease in men by 40 per cent, and reduces the risk of **dying** from CHD by 35 per cent.

See also Chapter 21.

GARLIC

In Germany, garlic tablets containing the equivalent of 4 g of fresh cloves are available on prescription to treat high blood cholesterol levels and high blood pressure.

In patients taking 800 mg dried garlic powder (e.g. Kwai tablets) per day, serum cholesterol levels fell by an average of 12 per cent after four months' therapy. Triglycerides (another form of fatty acid found in the blood) fell by up to 16 per cent.

Research suggests the active ingredient in garlic, allicin, prevents cells from taking up cholesterol and reduces cholesterol production in the liver.

Sulphur compounds formed by the degradation of allicin also contribute to garlic's beneficial effects. These sulphur compounds are incorporated into long-chain fatty acids, to act as antioxidants. This mechanism is particularly important in preventing CHD.

Garlic therapy also reduces average blood pressures by 8 per cent (systolic) and 12 per cent (diastolic) over a three-month period (*see* Chapter 12 on High Blood Pressure). This is thought to be due to dilation of blood vessels, and to garlic's beneficial effect on the way sodium and potassium ions cross cell membranes.

OILY FISH

Oily fish such as salmon, trout, mackerel, herring, salmon and sardines contain a fatty acid known as eicosapentanoic acid (EPA). This is processed in the body to make the blood less sticky, mainly by stopping blood platelet cells from clumping together. Eating oily fish regularly will lower the risk of CHD. If a heart attack does occur, EPA lowers the risk of dying from it. In men who have already had a heart attack, eating oily fish significantly reduces the chance of a second heart attack. If one does occur, the chances of dying from the second thrombosis are also decreased.

Dutch doctors have shown that men who eat fish once or twice a week can halve their risk of dying from a stroke. The average Western male should increase his weekly consumption of oily fish by a factor of 10 – to 300 g per week.

RED WINE

Red wine contains antioxidants that discourage atherosclerosis and decrease the stickiness of blood. It is especially beneficial if drunk while eating, when it neutralizes the effects of saturated fats in the diet.

FIBRE

Eating 3 g or more of soluble oat fibre (roughly equal to two large bowls of porridge) per day can lower total blood cholesterol levels by up to 0.16 mm/l. This is a small – but significant – change.

197

20 Tips to Help Avoid a Heart Attack

1   Stop smoking.
    Men who smoke are five times more likely to have a heart
    attack in their thirties and forties than non-smokers – and three
    times more likely to have one over all. Stopping smoking can
    reduce your risk of a heart attack by as much as 50 – 70 per
    cent within 5 years.

2   Lose any excess weight.
    Men who are overweight are one-and-a-half times more likely
    to have a heart attack than someone who maintains a healthy
    weight. If you are obese, your risk is doubled – especially if you
    store excess fat around your middle (apple shaped). Getting down
    to a healthy weight can reduce your risk of a heart attack by
    35 – 55 per cent.

3   Take regular exercise.
    Men who exercise for 20 – 30 minutes at least five times per
    week are half as likely to have a heart attack than those who
    are physically inactive. Activities such as DIY, gardening and
    dancing are just as effective as swimming or cycling for heart
    health.

4   Keep alcohol intake within safe limits.
    A moderate alcohol intake – especially of red wine – can reduce
    your risk of heart disease by 25 – 45 per cent. If you regularly
    drink more than 6 units in one session, however, your risk of a
    heart attack doubles. Men should aim to drink no more than 3
    – 4 units of alcohol per day, while women should drink no
    more than 2 – 3 units per day.
    1 unit of alcohol is equivalent to:
    – 100 ml (1 glass) of wine or
    – 50 ml (one measure) of sherry or
    – 25 ml (one tot) of spirits or
    – 300 ml (half a pint) of normal strength beer.

5   Watch the fats in your diet.
    One in three heart attacks are due to an unhealthy diet with
    too much fat and not enough starchy foods or fruit and vegeta-
    bles. The average man needs to reduce his fat intake by at least
    a quarter. Concentrate on obtaining beneficial fats such as
    olive, rapeseed, walnut, fish and evening primrose oils, and cut

back on fatty foods such as donuts, chips and cream. Choose reduced-fat foods where possible. Grill rather than fry. Eat red meat only once or twice a week and have more vegetarian meals instead.

6   Eat more carbohydrates.
Dietary carbohydrates should provide at least 55 – 60 per cent of daily calories. Eat more complex, unrefined carbohydrates such as wholegrain cereals, brown rice, wholemeal bread, wholewheat pasta and jacket potatoes while avoiding sugary foods. Men who eat a high carbohydrate diet are more likely to lose excess weight, lower their blood pressure and cholesterol levels, helping to avoid a heart attack.

7   Eat more fish.
Fish oils can thin the blood, lower blood pressure and – if you suffer from heart disease – can reduce your risk of a *fatal* heart attack by a third. The British Nutrition Foundation recommend increasing your consumption of oily fish (salmon, herrings, sardines, mackerel) to 300 g (3 portions) per week. If you don't like fish, consider taking an omega-3 fish oil supplement instead.

8   Eat at least five portions of fresh fruit and vegetables per day.
Fruit and vegetables contain important vitamins, minerals, antioxidants and beneficial plant hormones. Eating at least five servings per day reduces your risk of premature death from any cause at any age – especially from coronary heart disease – compared with those who eat less.

9   Eat more fibre.
Increasing the amount of fibre in your diet absorbs fats in the gut and slows their absorption so that your body handles them more easily. Eating 3 g or more of soluble oat fibre (roughly equal to two large bowls of porridge) every day has been shown to lower harmful blood cholesterol levels by a small by significant amount.

10   Cut back on salt.
Research suggests that at least one in two men are genetically programmed to develop high blood pressure if their intake of salt (sodium chloride) is excessive. Reducing salt intake from 9 g to 6 g (current UK Government recommendations) would lower your risk of a stroke by 22 per cent, prevent at least one

in seven heart attacks and your risk of death from CHD by 16 per cent. Unfortunately, around 75 per cent of dietary salt is hidden in processed foods including canned products, ready-prepared meals, biscuits, cakes and breakfast cereals. This means that without checking labels of bought products and avoiding those containing high amounts of salt, it is difficult to influence your salt intake as much as is desirable to reduce your risk of hypertension. Avoid obviously salty foods (crisps; bacon; pickled fish/meats; products tinned in brine) and stop adding salt during cooking or at the table. Obtain flavour from herbs, spices and black pepper instead. (N.B. A healthy intake of no more than 4 – 6 g salt per day is equivalent to 2 to 2.5 g sodium daily).

11   Avoid excess stress.
When you are under excess stress, your blood pressure goes up by an amount equivalent to carrying an extra 40 lb in weight, or an additional 20 years in age. Together with spasm of coronary arteries, this can trigger a heart attack. Take regular exercise (which burns off stress hormones) and take time out to relax whenever you feel tense. Stress-busting supplements such as ginseng will also help.

12   Have your blood pressure (BP) checked regularly.
High blood pressure affects one in five adults. It is known as the silent killer as it can creep up on you, without causing symptoms, to trigger a sudden heart attack or stroke. Even if your blood pressure is dangerously high, you may feel relatively well. Have your BP checked at least once a year. If your BP is high, good control will reduce your risk of a heart attack by 2 – 3 per cent for each 1-mm Hg fall in diastolic BP (the pressure in your system when your heart is relaxed between beats).

13   Have your urine checked regularly for glucose.
A man is two to three times more likely to have a heart attack if his blood sugar level is raised or poorly controlled. Have your urine screened regularly for glucose – at least once a year. If you have diabetes, you can reduce your risk of a heart attack by keeping your blood sugar level within tight limits – ask your doctor for further advice.

14   Have your blood fat levels checked.
Some types of fat in the circulation (for example HDL-choles-

terol) help to protect against a heart attack, while others (such as triglycerides, LDL-cholesterol) are linked with an increased risk of heart disease. If you are at risk of heart problems, your doctor will usually be happy to have your blood fat levels analysed. Reducing abnormally raised blood cholesterol levels by just 10 per cent could prevent one in four heart attacks occurring.

15   Consider taking garlic tablets.
Taking garlic tablets can lower high blood pressure, reduce high blood fat levels and thin the blood enough to reduce the risk of heart disease by up to 25 per cent. It has such a powerful effect that in Germany, garlic tablets containing the equivalent of 4 g of fresh cloves are available on prescription to treat high blood cholesterol levels and high blood pressure.

16   Consider taking an antioxidant supplement.
People with high blood levels of the antioxidant vitamins C and E (usually through taking supplements) are three times less likely to have a heart attack than those with low levels. It was also recently shown that taking high-dose vitamin E (400 iu or 268 mg) reduced the risk of a heart attack by a massive 75 per cent for men who already had heart disease. Antioxidant supplements are especially important for smokers and men with diabetes.

17   Consider taking a folic acid supplement.
Around one in 10 men have inherited high blood levels of the amino acid, homocysteine. This damages artery linings and more than triples the risk of a heart attack. One in 160,000 people have extremely high levels with 30 times the risk of premature heart disease. High levels of homocysteine can be reduced by taking supplements of folic acid (400–650 mcg per day). Vitamins B_6 and B_{12} also have a beneficial effect. Foods rich in folic acid include green leafy vegetables (such as spinach, broccoli, Brussel sprouts) and whole grains.

18   Consider taking half an aspirin a day.
Aspirin is so powerful at preventing blood clots that only half a tablet (150 mg) is needed per day to reduce your risk of a heart attack by a third. You may benefit from taking aspirin if you have:

angina
already had a heart attack
had heart surgery
poor circulation in the limbs
diabetes
an increased risk of heart disease from any cause.
Ask your doctor for further advice.

19 Drink more tea!
Research suggests that drinking four cups of tea per day – 1,460 cups per year – may halve your risk of a heart attack. Tea is a rich source of flavonoids – the chemicals known to give red wine its beneficial properties. Other important sources of flavonoids include garlic, onions and apples.

20 Adopt a positive attitude to life.
Men who smile, laugh and think positively are less likely to have a heart attack than those with a negative outlook on life. Thinking positive has also been shown to boost immunity and reduce the risk of infections. Men who laugh regularly seem to be healthier over all, and have less infections than those eaten up with anger and hostility.

12

HIGH BLOOD PRESSURE

High blood pressure, or hypertension, affects around 20 per cent of the adult male population. It is known as the silent killer as it creeps up without symptoms to cause a sudden heart attack or stroke. Even if your blood pressure is dangerously high, you may feel relatively well.

Blood pressure (BP) is gauged according to how much mercury (measured in a column length) it can support. Blood pressure is therefore expressed in millimetres of mercury (mmHg). BP is highest as blood surges through the system when the heart pumps. It is lowest as the heart relaxes between beats. BP is recorded as the higher (systolic) pressure over the lower (diastolic) reading. A typical 20-year-old might have a BP of 120/70 mmHg. A fit 50-year-old might have a BP of around 150/85 mmHg.

The World Health Organization defines hypertension as a blood pressure that is consistently greater than 160 mmHg (systolic) and 95 mmHg (diastolic). Systolic blood pressures of 140–160 mmHg and diastolic values of 90–95 mmHg are referred to as mild, or borderline hypertension. A 50-year-old man with untreated hypertension might have a BP of 180/100 mmHg or higher.

The best analogy to explain how hypertension develops is to compare circulating blood with water running through a hose pipe. Water pressure within a hose pipe can be raised by increasing the power of the pump (tap) or by squeezing the pipe and reducing its diameter. In exactly the same way, blood pressure can be increased within the circulation by increasing the work of the heart or by reducing the diameter of the vessels through which the blood flows.

BP varies enormously – by as much as 70 mmHg – throughout the day. Lowest values are recorded during sleep, around three to four hours after the person has fallen to sleep. Highest levels naturally occur at around midday, or whenever the person in question has been awake for about four hours. Physical exercise such as climbing stairs or riding a bicycle temporarily increase BP, but this is an entirely normal physiological response.

Two male activities in particular can produce phenomenally high BPs. These are weight lifting and sexual intercourse. Since these are transient effects, they do not seem to cause any harm.

Emotions such as anger also raise BP. This is because adrenaline and other stress hormones stimulate constriction of the blood vessels and also get the heart pumping faster.

WHAT CAUSES HIGH BP?

High BP results from interactions between inherited, developmental and lifestyle factors. There are probably several abnormal genes involved in high BP, which alone or in combination can cause high BP in later life.

Events that occur during foetal development prior to birth can also programme in a tendency to develop hypertension, stroke or a heart attack. This is probably due to impaired maternal nutrition affecting arterial development. Research shows that low birth weight babies are more likely to develop high BP as adults. Average adult systolic BP increases by 11 mmHg as birth weight goes down from 7.5 lb to 5.5 lb. The size of the placenta at birth is also important. Average systolic BP rises by 15 mmHg as placental weight increases from 1 lb to 1.5 lb in weight. The highest BPs therefore occur in men who were born small babies with large placentas. This may be due to abnormal arterial and blood circulatory patterns being laid down as a result of imbalances between the placenta and the baby.

This is borne out by research that links fingerprint patterns with the risk of developing high BP in later life. Fingerprints are laid down in the womb in the first few weeks following conception. Their patterns are linked to the degree of bumpiness and swelling of the developing fingertips, which in turn is related to irregular blood circulation.

Fingerprint patterns take the form of arches, loops or whorls *(see Figure 18, below)*. The more whorls you have, the more likely you are to become hypertensive. Researchers have found that people with at least one whorl have a BP that is 6 per cent higher than people with no whorls. BP then generally increases as the number of whorls increases. The maximum number of whorls is 10 (two per digit). The average number tends to be two or three.

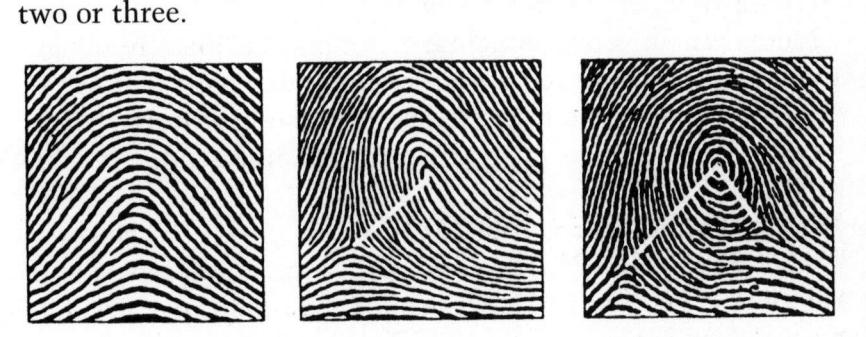

Figure 18: Fingertip whorls and hypertension

On top of these genetic and developmental predispositions, environmental factors interact to produce hypertension.

It is now thought that the rise in BP with increasing age that is commonly seen in Western countries is linked with our lifetime intake of salt. The chemical name for salt is sodium chloride. It is the sodium that is linked with high BP – the average male sodium consumption in the UK is around 3.5 g per day, which is far too high *(see Chapter 20)*. Some men eat twice this amount and are sitting ducks for hypertension.

Obesity is also linked with hypertension in some people, possibly because the heart has to pump harder to get blood around a larger body. Fat people are also more likely to have a high saturated fat diet, high blood cholesterol levels and a greater amount of furring up and narrowing of the arteries *(see Chapters 11 and 17)*.

Another important environmental factor is alcohol intake. Men who regularly drink more than three units of alcohol per day *(see page 280)* tend to have higher BPs. Many men drink more than this and have normal BP – it depends upon your underlying genes.

The other major environmental factor linked with high BP is stress. Exposure to stress seems to make part of the nervous system overactive in some people, leading to hypertension. Stress leads to increased circulating levels of adrenaline and overactivity of the sympathetic nervous system. This triggers arterial spasm and hypertension.

More than one environmental factor may be operative at any one time. It seems that a man exposed to excess salt at the same time he is feeling stressed is more likely to develop high BP than a man who is just exposed to too much salt, or who is just under stress *(see Chapter 17)*.

Hypertension needs to be taken seriously. It is a powerful predictor of a number of diseases that are common causes of ill health and death in males from middle age onwards. The two commonest consequences of high BP are heart attacks and strokes.

As hypertension makes it more difficult for the heart to pump blood out against the pressure resistance, it also leads to thickening of heart muscle and dilation of the heart chambers. The heart may become a floppy, dilated bag of muscle which is unable to pump efficiently. This leads to heart failure, with fluid accumulating within the body. Thickened heart muscle will also outgrow its blood supply, to result in angina pain.

High BP damages the inside lining of arteries throughout the body. This damage triggers the accumulation of fatty plaques and thrombosis (clots) which may eventually completely block blood flow. Tissues that are cut off from blood and oxygen rapidly die and this can lead to a heart attack (myocardial infarction) or a stroke. It is estimated that, for a man in his forties, each rise of 10 mm Hg in systolic BP increases the risk of heart disease by a massive 20 per cent.

High BP can also cause the equivalent of a blow-out in delicate blood vessels in the brain. This leads to another type of stroke in which haemorrhaging occurs, rather than death of brain cells due to blockage of blood vessels with a clot.

Small blood vessels within the body are even more vulnerable to the effects of high BP than larger arteries. Damage to small blood vessels at the back of the eye leads to retinal haemorrhages and visual disturbances. The eye acts like a window onto the brain, and any small vessel damage seen here mimics the changes happening inside the brain that might lead to a stroke.

Damage to small blood vessels in the kidney interferes with the production of urine, so fluid starts to accumulate in the body. This form of kidney failure is now relatively uncommon because drug treatment to control hypertension prevents it.

HOW TO PREVENT OR REDUCE HIGH BP

You cannot do much to alter your genes (yet) or reprogramme your foetal development. What you can do is alter your lifestyle to minimize the risk of developing hypertension in later life. If you already have high BP, whether it is raised severely, slightly or only moderately, you must reduce your exposure to environmental factors that will inevitably make it worse.

Lifestyle changes that can help prevent or treat high BP include:

cutting right back on salt intake: do not add salt at the table or during cooking; avoid salty foods such as crisps; bacon;

tinned, cured, smoked, or pickled fish/meats; meat paste; paté; ready prepared meals; tinned vegetables or tuna in brine; tinned or packet soups, sauces, stock cubes and yeast extracts.

By not adding salt at the table, by reducing the amount of salt used during cooking and by avoiding salty foods you can cut systolic BP by at least 5 mmHg. If everyone did this, it is estimated that the incidence of stroke in the population would be reduced by 26 per cent, and that of coronary heart disease by 15 per cent.

Salt is easily replaceable with spices. It does not take long to retrain your taste buds. Ensuring you eat plenty of potassium-rich foods will also help. Potassium ions are linked with sodium ions in the body. The kidney swaps potassium for sodium in the urine, so the more potassium you eat the more sodium you excrete. Too much potassium can, unfortunately, be harmful as well, so the best way to ensure adequate but safe supplies is to eat potassium-rich foods. These include all fruit, especially bananas, dried apricots, fruit juices and fruit yoghurts; all vegetables, especially pulses, mushrooms, potatoes and spinach; wholegrain breakfast cereals and, surprisingly, coffee.

Small amounts of potassium salts (Ruthmol, Selora) are also useful as sodium replacements but they can be a little bitter. Go easy on them as too much potassium causes problems of its own.

- Cut back on alcohol intake if this is excessive. Keep within the 21 units per week maximum for males. If you can, drop back to 14 units per week or less. (See page 280 for definitions of units of alcohol.)
- Lose any excess weight through a combination of diet and exercise. Exercise lasting for at least 20 minutes three times per week can in itself lower high BP. You need to increase your pulse rate to around 110–120 per minute and work up a light sweat.
- At the same time, men who smoke should stop. High BP and smoking together damage blood vessels even faster than would be expected from either alone. This will almost certainly lead

to coronary heart disease in the future.

- If your cholesterol levels are harmfully raised, you should also cut back on your intake of saturated (animal) fat. This contributes to furring up and narrowing of arteries and will lead inexorably to coronary heart disease *(see Chapter 11)*.

If despite these lifestyle changes your BP consistently remains high, you will need treatment with drugs. These are essential to control your BP and minimize your risk of a heart attack, stroke, heart failure, kidney failure and other problems related to vascular damage.

The aim of anti-hypertensive treatment is to reduce diastolic BP to below 90 mmHg and/or to reduce systolic BP to below 160 mmHg.

The main drugs now used to treat hypertension are:

DIURETICS (WATER TABLETS)

Diuretics lower BP by decreasing the amount of fluid within the circulation. They also cause mild dilation of small arteries.

BETA-BLOCKERS

These drugs damp down nerve pathways that cause blood vessel constriction. They slow the heart rate and reduce the force of contraction of the heart.

CALCIUM CHANNEL ANTAGONISTS

These drugs block the movement of calcium ions through cell membranes. This lowers BP by relaxing muscles in arterial walls, and by reducing the force of contraction of the heart.

ACE INHIBITORS

These block formation of Angiotensin Converting Enzyme (ACE). Ace is a powerful constrictor of blood vessels, so blocking it leads to blood vessel dilation. ACE inhibitors also increase blood flow to the kidneys, so more fluid is lost as urine.

ALPHA ANTAGONISTS

These drugs lower BP by dilating arteries and veins.

ANGIOTENSIN II ANTAGONISTS

This new class of drug has only recently become available. They dilate blood vessels, stimulate kidney function and may also have a direct action on the brain to reduce drinking and increase urine output.

As hypertension is common, it is worth having your BP checked on a regular basis. Early diagnosis, lifestyle changes and the prescription of necessary drugs can control BP and save many lives.

Every male should have his BP checked at least once before the age of 30 years. Over the age of 30, BP should be checked at least once every five years – preferably every one to two years.

13

CANCER

Cancer is one of the most common causes of death in males aged 15 to 64, and unfortunately it is on the increase.

One in three will suffer a cancer at some stage during his life, and one in four men will die from it. The commonest male cancers in the Western world are those that affect the:

- lungs
- skin (non-melanoma)
- colon and rectum
- prostate
- bladder
- stomach
- lymphatic system (Non-Hodgkin's lymphoma)
- pancreas
- oesophagus
- white blood cells (Leukaemia).

Worldwide, lung cancer is the commonest male tumour, having recently overtaken cancer of the stomach. Unfortunately, the overall incidence of all tumours seems to be rising. One study in Sweden, for example, has shown that over the last 30 years the incidence of cancer has risen by 55 per cent in men over the age of 50. For men under the age of 30, the incidence of cancer had increased by up to 40 per cent. It seems that the rise in incidence of cancer is linked with increased exposure to environmental carcinogens and ionizing radiation. Some cancers are already linked with particular causative agents:

- Smoking is associated with 90 per cent of lung cancers and a third of all other cancer deaths.
- Occupation is linked with one in 10 lung cancers: cranemen, derrickmen and hoistmen have a 14-fold increased risk of lung cancer, while sheet metal workers, tinsmiths, bookbinders and printing trade workers have three times the normal risk.
- Alcohol is linked with cancer of the tongue, throat, oesophagus and liver.
- Occupational exposure to certain chemicals is linked with cancer of the scrotum (*see page 42*)
- A poor diet (low in antioxidant vitamins and fibre and high in saturated fat) is linked with over a third of all malignancies.
- Some cancers have an hereditary link, for example cancer of the prostate gland and testes.

The good news is that cancer detection and treatment are two of the fastest growing fields in medicine, and many cancers are now curable if caught at an early stage. With new gene therapy techniques it is hoped that tumour cells can be 'switched off' or made more visible to the immune system for targeted eradication.

WARNING SIGNS FOR THE EARLY DIAGNOSIS OF CANCER

There are several warning signs to look out for that might indicate you have a tumour. Although in many cases these signs will be due to something less sinister, it is better to worry, get checked and receive an all clear than to dismiss the signs and delay an important diagnosis. The signs to watch out for include:

- weight loss for no apparent reason
- loss of appetite with tiredness and listlessness
- a scab, sore or ulcer that does not heal within three weeks
- a mole or other skin blemish that enlarges, crusts, bleeds, itches or becomes darker in colour
- a persistent, nagging cough
- coughing up blood
- a change in bowel habit
- a change in bladder habit
- blood in the urine
- blood or brown 'coffee grounds' in vomit
- difficulty swallowing
- feeling full despite eating very little
- hoarseness lasting more than three weeks
- a persistent sore throat
- unusual bleeding or discharge from any orifice
- unusual thickening or a lump anywhere on the body
- a change in the shape or size of the testes
- nagging indigestion that keeps coming back
- persistent abdominal pain
- black bowel motions
- severe, recurrent headaches
- recurrent deep pain in any part of the body.

CANCER PREVENTION

Many cancers can be prevented by altering your diet and lifestyle. You can significantly reduce your risk of developing the disease by:

- giving up smoking
- losing excess weight and taking regular exercise
- reducing exposure to sun and ultra-violet (UV) irradiation
- using high-factor sun screens and covering up whenever you are

exposed to the sun
- avoiding sunburn
- obeying safety rules and wearing protective clothing when working with dangerous chemicals or irradiation processes
- avoiding skin exposure to soot, tar, mineral oils and other noxious substances
- keeping alcohol intake within safe limits
- avoiding sexually transmissible diseases by practising safer sex
- examining your testicles regularly once per month
- washing under the foreskin regularly
- eating a high-fibre diet and avoiding constipation
- following a diet low in saturated fats
- eating a diet rich in vitamins C, E and betacarotene
- eating at least five portions of fruit and vegetables per day
- increasing your intake of wholegrain cereals and pulses
- reducing your intake of salt-cured, salt-pickled and smoked foods

In fact, a diet that is good for the heart is also excellent at reducing the risk of cancer *(see page 274)*.

See also the chapters that discuss specific male cancers *(Chapters 1, 2, 6, 10, 16 and 17)*.

14

THE MALE INTESTINAL TRACT

Indigestion and peptic ulcers affect twice as many men as women, with over 60 per cent of the adult male population suffering symptoms at some time during their lives.

Indigestion is a common term covering a variety of symptoms related to eating. These include feelings of distension from swallowing air, flatulence from excessive wind in the intestines, nausea, abdominal pain and sensations of burning due to acid reflux.

GASTRO-OESOPHAGEAL REFLUX DISEASE

Gastro-oesophageal reflux disease (GORD) is due to acidic stomach contents refluxing up into the oesophagus – the tube connecting the mouth and stomach. Normally this reflux is prevented by a muscle sphincter and by a downward-propelling action of the oesophageal muscles. If, however, muscle action is uncoordinated, if a hiatus hernia is present, or if the stomach is excessively full, reflux can occur.

The main symptom of GORD is heartburn. This hot,

burning sensation is felt behind the sternum and may rise up into the throat. It usually comes on within 30 minutes of eating a meal and may be precipitated by exercise or by bending or lying down, especially after eating. Meals containing fat, pastry, chocolate, peppermint, fruit juices, coffee or alcohol frequently trigger attacks.

In men under the age of 40, antacids, prokinetic agents (which co-ordinate muscle contraction) and drugs that damp down acid secretions (e.g. cimetidine, ranitidine) are used to damp down symptoms.

In men over the age of 40, or for those with more sinister symptoms (weight loss, difficulty swallowing, vomiting, bleeding, anaemia, early feelings of fullness, severe pain), further investigation is required to eliminate the possibility of a peptic ulcer or stomach cancer.

TIPS TO ALLEVIATE THE SYMPTOMS OF GORD

- Lose any excess weight.
- If you smoke, stop or cut down.
- Eat little and often throughout the day, rather than the traditional three large meals.
- Avoid drinking large quantities of liquid at any one time.
- Avoid hot, acid, spicy, fatty foods.
- Avoid peppermint, chocolate and fruit juices.
- Avoid tea and coffee.
- Cut back on alcohol intake.
- Avoid aspirin and related drugs – use paracetamol.
- Avoid stooping, bending or lying down after eating.
- Avoid late-night eating.
- Elevate the head of your bed by about 15–20 cm (6–8 in).
- Wear loose clothing.
- Drinking a glass of milk may ease your symptoms.
- If you feel blown out with wind, take a teaspoon of bicarbonate of soda dissolved in a glass of warm water every hour for up to three hours – but do not take any more than this.

NB Losing weight and giving up smoking are the two most useful measures for reducing gastro-oesophageal reflux.

If you suffer from recurrent indigestion, it is important to tell your doctor. A recent Gallup poll of over 1,000 people found that within the past 12 months 48 per cent had suffered heartburn but that only 25 per cent had sought help.

If you have tried over-the-counter antacids and they haven't controlled your symptoms, you should also tell this to the doctor, otherwise you may end up with a similar preparation instead of something stronger. This is important, as it has been found that taking antacids does not protect against the damage done by acid on delicate stomach and intestinal tissues. After 10–20 years, scarring (and a resulting difficulty swallowing) can occur. One in 10 people taking regular antacids could have a serious underlying problem, so always consult a doctor.

GASTRITIS

The stomach is normally protected from digesting itself by a lining of mucus. If this mucus mantle is eroded, however, inflammation of the stomach wall can occur. Gastritis produces symptoms similar to those of a stomach ulcer: burning or gnawing pain in the upper abdomen, nausea and vomiting. If gastritis is severe, there may be blood in the vomit (haematemesis). The blood is usually partly digested and clotted, so that is resembles dark brown coffee grounds in the vomit.

Acute gastritis can be triggered by substances that irritate the stomach lining, such as cigarettes, alcohol, aspirin, ibuprofen and other non-steroidal anti-inflammatory analgesic drugs.

Helicobacter pylori

The primary cause of gastritis is now known to be infection of the stomach with a bacterium called *Helicobacter pylori*. In the UK, at least 20 per cent of 30-year-old men and 50 per cent of those over the age of 50 are infected. In some parts of the world such as in South America and Africa, colonization rates are higher, with up to 90 per cent of 20 year olds infected.

217

Helicobacter pylori is a motile bacterium that burrows into the mucous lining of the stomach and exposes the stomach wall to acid attack. It can survive the high concentrations of acid by producing an enzyme (urease) which converts small quantities of urea into a bubble of ammonia gas. This alkaline bubble coats the bacterium and protects it from stomach acids. At the same time, the ammonia acts as another irritant to inflame the stomach wall.

Helicobacter pylori can be tested for in a number of ways:

* blood tests to look for antibodies to the bacteria
* breath tests – the patient swallows some radioactive urea, then half an hour later breathes into a sealed bag. If Helicobacter is present, its enzyme will convert urea to ammonia, so that radioactive ammonia will be detected in the bag.
* a new non-invasive test picks up signs of infection from saliva

Once diagnosed, Helicobacter can be eradicated by a mixture of two antibiotics plus bismuth (triple therapy) or one antibiotic plus a drug that stops the stomach from making acid (double therapy). Unfortunately this treatment (especially triple therapy) is unpleasant with side-effects of a sore mouth, a disagreeable metallic after-taste left in the mouth, nausea, diarrhoea, abdominal pain and blackening of the stools and tongue. One in five patients drops out of treatment with triple therapy; double therapy is better tolerated.

New research from New Zealand suggests that honey made from the flower of the Manuka, or New Zealand Tea Tree, contains a unique antibiotic that can also eradicate Helicobacter. Taking four teaspoons of Manuka honey four times per day on an empty stomach for eight weeks can eradicate infection. Manuka honey is available in some healthfood shops.

NB Men with diabetes should consult their doctor before using honey treatments.

Peptic Ulcers

Peptic ulcers affect twice as many men as women, and in the UK one in 30 adults suffers at some stage during his or her life. Duodenal ulcers (affecting the duodenum – the tube that leads out of the stomach) are more common, affecting around one in 10 adults. The peak age for developing a duodenal ulcer is 20–40 years. Gastric ulcers tend to occur 10–20 years later.

In the UK, it is estimated that in any one year up to a million people suffer a peptic ulcer. Ninety per cent of these are recurrent ulcers.

Helicobacter pylori infection is associated with 85 per cent of gastric ulcers and virtually all duodenal ulcers. The increasing recognition and treatment of this important infection has resulted in the incidence and recurrence rates of peptic ulcers starting to fall.

Peptic ulcers typically produce symptoms of:

- gnawing, localized pain
- pain at night
- pain that is relieved by antacids
- pain that is relieved by vomiting
- pain that (in the case of stomach ulcers) may be exacerbated by eating
- pain that (in the case of duodenal) ulcers may be relieved by eating

In men under the age of 40, a trial of anti-ulcer treatment is usually given to see if symptoms improve. Smoking and aspirin-related drugs should be stopped as these may have triggered the problem in the first place. If symptoms recur after treatment, investigation is essential to confirm the diagnosis and to rule out the possibility of stomach cancer.

In men over the age of 40 years, investigation is necessary before anti-ulcer treatment is started. Antacids can be used to relieve symptoms while awaiting the results of this investigation.

The most usual modern investigation of peptic pain is

endoscopy. A light sedative is given into a vein to relax you and to minimize discomfort. A thin, flexible tube is then passed down into the stomach through the mouth. This tube contains a light, a magnified viewing system and biopsy forceps. It allows visual inspection of the lining of the stomach and duodenum and will identify areas of inflammation (gastritis), ulceration, bleeding and scarring. Suspicious areas can be biopsied (a small sample taken out) and examined so that the possibility of malignancy can be ruled out.

Although you are awake throughout an endoscopy, most patients do not remember it afterwards because of the sedative they are given.

Treatment

There are several different treatments for peptic ulcers. Self-help measures include giving up smoking, avoiding alcohol, tea and coffee, aspirin and related drugs such as ibuprofen, and eating several small meals per day rather than three larger ones. Other simple treatments include:

- antacids (e.g. aluminium hydroxide, calcium carbonate, magnesium salts, sodium bicarbonate), which neutralize excess acidity
- H_2 blockers (e.g. ranitidine, cimetidine, famotidine, nizatidine), which reduce acid secretion by blocking the receptors on acid-producing cells. These heal up to 85 per cent of ulcers within two months. Around 80 per cent of ulcers will recur within a year of stopping treatment, however, so long-term maintenance therapy is used for some patients.
- proton pump inhibitors (e.g. omeprazole), which stop acid secretion and promote more rapid ulcer healing than H_2 blockers. Ninety per cent of ulcers are healed within one month, but again, relapse is common once treatment has stopped.
- Cytoprotectants (e.g. sucralfate, carbenoxolone, misoprostol), which either increase mucus secretion in the stomach or coat the ulcer to act as a barrier to acid.
- Helicobacter eradication therapy (see page 218). Only 1–2 per cent

of patients have recurrent peptic ulceration following this procedure.

Complications

If a peptic ulcer erodes a blood vessel, bleeding results. If bleeding is low key and recurrent, iron-deficiency anaemia can result, with progressive tiredness, pallor and even shortness of breath. More usually, bleeding is due to erosion of an artery, which can produce sudden, severe haemorrhage. Nausea and vomiting occur, with either bright red or semi-digested blood in the vomit which resembles coffee grounds. Digested blood that continues down the intestinal tract produces foul-smelling, tarry black bowel motions.

Rarely, a peptic ulcer may perforate the wall of the digestive tract. Irritant intestinal secretions full of acids and enzymes leak into the abdominal cavity to produce severe inflammation and pain due to peritonitis.

Chronic ulceration can produce scarring of the exit from the stomach and the duodenum. This causes narrowing in the passages and obstructs the downward course of food, resulting in vomiting and weight loss.

All peptic ulcer complications require urgent admission to hospital for emergency treatment which usually involves surgery.

Contact a doctor for advice if:

- your pain is very severe
- any abdominal pain lasts more than four hours, especially if it starts to get worse
- prolonged vomiting occurs
- you vomit blood, brown-stained liquid or what looks like brown coffee grounds
- you start to pass very dark or black bowel motions
- you feel very weak or faint.

IRRITABLE BOWEL SYNDROME

Irritable bowel syndrome (IBS) affects at least a quarter of the population. Although only one in three sufferers is male, this still represents a sizable proportion of the adult male population – around one in 12. Symptoms usually begin between the ages of 15 and 40 but it can affect anyone at any age. It is also known as irritable colon, spastic colon or mucous colitis.

The cause of IBS is not understood. The basic problem is a disturbance of muscle contraction in the intestinal tract, but no physical abnormality has yet been found as its cause.

The intestines are a long muscular tube which contracts in ordered waves. This propels food along while nutrients and water are absorbed. In irritable bowel syndrome, these contractions are uncoordinated and cramps occur. Nobody yet knows why.

The main symptoms of IBS are pain, wind, bloating, distension, sensations of incompletely evacuating the bowels, increased mucus from the back passage, and constipation or diarrhoea (or bouts of each).

As these symptoms also occur in more serious bowel conditions it is important to have them checked by your doctor – you should never make a diagnosis of IBS yourself. Most importantly, if you notice any change in your usual bowel habit, any blood or blackness in your stools, or weight loss, seek urgent medical advice.

The pain of IBS is cramp-like or colicky and comes and goes in waves. It is felt anywhere in the abdomen but is often worse on the lower left-hand side. The pain may worsen after eating as this stimulates contraction of the colon (gastrocolic reflex). Sufferers usually find that opening the bowels or passing wind brings relief.

Wind is a common problem. Because the bowels are not contracting properly, air that is naturally swallowed when eating and drinking builds up. It burbles around causing pain, distension and noises (borborygmi) until escaping suddenly and sometimes explosively.

Constipation is another common feature of IBS, as spasm of

the muscular bowel walls squashes its contents rather than pushing them through. As a result the bowels may not open for days at a time. When they do, straining is necessary to push out hard, rabbity pellets or thin ribbons of faeces.

The bowels also frequently work overtime, with increased mucus secretion and intestinal hurry (diarrhoea). Constipation and diarrhoea often alternate and sufferers may notice an unpleasant sensation of not completely evacuating the bowels.

At present, IBS is a diagnosis of exclusion, there is no definitive test that can pick it up. Initial examination of the abdomen is performed to elicit areas of tenderness and check for obvious lumps. A digital rectal examination is mandatory for any bowel problem. This is only slightly uncomfortable and gives important information regarding the texture of the bowel lining and whether the rectum is full or empty of stool, and can enable the detection of rectal tumours.

Blood tests may be taken to look for anaemia, thyroid problems and signs of infection or inflammation. Further investigation of the lower bowel involves a barium enema, or endoscopy in which a scope is passed into the rectum and lower (sigmoid) colon. If a higher part of the bowel is examined via colonoscopy, light sedation is given. (A colonoscopy is a procedure in which a viewing device is inserted into the back passage so that the large colon can be examined and biopsied.)

Treatment

Once more serious conditions such as bowel tumours or inflammatory bowel disease are ruled out, the treatment of IBS is aimed at controlling symptoms. Unfortunately, as yet there is no cure. Controlling the symptoms involves:

- antispasmodics (e.g. alverine, mebeverine, peppermint oil) to relax the bowel and dampen painful spasms
- peppermint capsules to prevent wind distention
- following a high-fibre diet and taking bulking agents (e.g. bran, methylcellulose)

- anti-diarrhoeal agents (e.g. loperamide) to relieve bowel looseness.

In up to a quarter of men, a high-fibre diet initially makes the bloating and distension of IBS worse. This effect disappears after two or three weeks, however, so it is important to persevere. The bloating may be related to not drinking enough fluids. Bulking agents usually come in the form of granules which are taken once or twice a day with plenty of water. The fibre swells up in the bowel and provides bulk for the intestines to grip. This helps propel waste through efficiently.

The diarrhoea associated with IBS is often worse in the first few hours of waking. In this case, an anti-diarrhoeal drug such as loperamide is best taken last thing before bed and again after the first bowel action of the day. Treatment should only be used for short periods of time without the advice of your doctor. It is also worth avoiding fruit juices and prunes and cutting down on milk and dairy products if your bowels are very loose.

Self-help Tips

There are many dietary and lifestyle changes you can make to help your symptoms:

- Cut out all prepacked or processed foods and stick to a natural, whole food diet
- Eat a high-fibre diet containing wholegrain bread, wholemeal pasta, brown rice and unsweetened wholegrain breakfast cereals such as muesli (granola) or porridge. Some people find this makes their symptoms worse, but persevere for three to four weeks before deciding this is not working for you.
- Fresh fruit and vegetables – especially nuts, seeds, figs, apricots, prunes, peas, sweetcorn and beans – are especially high in fibre.
- Cut down on the amount of saturated fat in your diet. Avoid dairy products such as butter, cream and whole-fat milk. Instead, try semi-skimmed or skimmed milk, and olive-oil based products in place of butter. Low-fat fromage frais is a delicious and healthy substitute for cream.

- Many people find that live bio-yoghurt containing a culture of the bacterium *Lactobacillus acidophilus* relieves their symptoms. Lactobacilli are able to colonize the bowel and this may help damp down symptoms.
- Try avoiding red meat and see if this improves your symptoms. Eat more fish and skinless white meat in its place.
- Avoid sugar, cakes, sweets and chocolate.
- Do not fry or roast your food, – grill, bake, casserole or steam instead.
- Many natural herbs and spices contain substances that calm the bowels, relieve spasm and prevent a build-up of wind. These include aniseed, chamomile, lemon balm, clove, dill, fennel, black pepper, marjoram, parsley, peppermint, rosemary and spearmint. Use them as a garnish on food or as soothing, herbal teas. Plain infusions of chamomile or peppermint are available, as are delicious combinations such as chamomile and spearmint or fennel and lemon balm.
- Stop smoking and avoid passive smoking, too. There are receptors in the intestinal tract which react with nicotine and cause the bowel to constrict, making symptoms worse.
- Increase the amount of exercise you take. This hastens bowel emptying and can relieve bloating and distension. For those who are immobile, abdominal massage is an alternative.
- Try to avoid unnecessary stress. The bowel contains receptors that interact with stress hormones, which will make spasm and diarrhoea worse.

Many alternative treatments can help to relieve IBS. They include acupuncture, homoeopathy, floatation therapy and hypnotherapy.

At present there is no cure for IBS, but research is ongoing and may provide answers in the future. For example, it was recently found that patients who had an operation for haemorrhoids also noticed a significant improvement in their symptoms of IBS. This might be due to the cutting of small nerves which prevented feedback hyperstimulation of the intestines.

HAEMORRHOIDS

Haemorrhoids (piles) are surprisingly common, with up to 40 per cent of adult males affected. A pile is a swollen varicose vein in the back passage (rectum). Haemorrhoids are frequently multiple and, if they occur close to the anal opening, can protrude to form external piles. If they occur higher up, so they are hidden from view, they are known as internal piles.

External piles tend to be dark red or purple in colour as they are covered by a thick layer of skin. Internal piles are lined by a mucous membrane and are therefore bright red, shiny and moist.

Haemorrhoids form because our rectal veins are the lowest in the system carrying blood from the liver to the heart. This means an enormous weight of blood bears down on them due to the effects of gravity. This causes stretching of the veins and rupturing of their containing tissues, especially if you spend long periods of time standing on your feet. Piles can also be hereditary and associated with congenital weakness of veins in the back passage. Any increase in pressure such as straining from constipation will also cause them to expand. In fact, the commonest cause of piles is long-term constipation due to lack of fibre in the diet.

The symptoms commonly associated with piles are:

- bleeding from the back passage – usually bright red blood
- dull, dragging aching sensations in the back passage
- pain, especially on opening your bowels
- mucous discharge
- itching.

You should not diagnose piles yourself as many of their symptoms are similar to those of more serious diseases such as inflammatory bowel disease or even cancer. Always consult a doctor, especially if you notice blood either in or on your motions.

Treatment

Mild haemorrhoids are helped by drinking plenty of fluids and eating a high-fibre diet. This keeps bowel movements regular and soft and avoids straining.

It is important to get into a regular routine of opening your bowels at least once per day. But never strain hard or you will make your piles worse. Leaning forward from the hips while sitting on the toilet will help to reduce straining.

- Always go to the toilet when you first feel the need – do not delay opening your bowels however busy you are.
- The area around the anus should be cleaned with unperfumed soap and warm water after every bowel movement. This prevents infection and encourages healing. A bidet is ideal. Pat yourself dry with absorbent tissue or use a hairdryer rather than rubbing the area with a towel.
- Keep your bottom as dry as possible. Cotton underwear is more absorbent than nylon. Many people also keep a tissue or cotton wool (changed frequently) between their buttocks. But this may rub, so do be careful.
- Rectal suppositories and creams are soothing. These contain local anaesthetics and drugs which damp down inflammation, itching, swelling and pain. Some of the best ones are only available on prescription.
- Take regular exercise to encourage a healthier circulation, and lose any excess weight.
- If you get a bad attack of pain and discomfort, raise the foot of your bed by 15–20 cm (6–8 in) and lie down so your feet are higher than your head. Gravity will then help blood drain away from your haemorrhoids. External piles can be gently pushed back using the fingers and plenty of soothing, lubricating cream, but don't press too hard.

Sometimes blood becomes trapped inside an external pile and starts to clot. The pile is then said to have strangulated, causing intense pain. Instant relief can be obtained by a doctor anaesthetizing the pile with local anaesthetic cream, and then making a small incision to shell out the clotted blood.

When haemorrhoids are bad enough to interfere with your daily life, it is best to have something permanent done about them. Piles can be:

- sealed off with a sclerosant injection
- shrivelled with a freezing cryoprobe
- tied off with a tight elastic band. Banding is painless and no anaesthetic is needed. The procedure cuts off the blood supply to the haemorrhoid, which then withers and drops off painlessly within a few days.
- removed under general anaesthetic via a haemorrhoidectomy operation. The piles are cut away, together with some of the rectal wall lining, and sutured. Unfortunately, this operation is quite painful and you will need strong painkillers and laxatives to see you through the first few days after surgery. Hospitalization is necessary until you can open your bowels easily. Complete healing takes three to six weeks.

HERNIAS

A hernia is the name given to any organ or tissue that protrudes through a weakness in the parts that normally contain it. The most common hernias involve the intestine, which can protrude through a weakness in the abdominal wall. This weakness may be:

- a normal anatomical weakness found in everyone (e.g. the inguinal canal; the belly button)
- an abnormal weakness caused by a congenital defect or acquired as a result of injury or disease.

Acquired weaknesses often result from straining (e.g. when lifting heavy objects, coughing, being constipated), abdominal surgery, or through the laying down of fat in the overweight.

In the UK, over 80,000 hernia repair operations (herniorrhaphy or hernioplasty) are carried out each year. Of these, around 10,000 are to repair a hernia that has recurred after previous surgery.

Men are 12 times more likely to develop a hernia than women and, overall, 3 per cent of adult males will eventually have a hernia repair. This is mainly because of the weakness opened up by the testes descending into the scrotum during development *(see pages 27 and 230)*. Another factor is the straining due to manual labouring jobs.

The important things your doctor needs to work out about any hernia is whether the bowel loop can be popped back into its normal place *(reducible)*, whether it is trapped *(irreducible)* or whether its blood supply is in danger *(strangulated)*.

A *reducible* hernia simply presents as a lump which is painless and often disappears when the person affected lies down. With a little gentle encouragement the lump can be massaged back into the abdomen. On coughing, it will protrude again and, if a hand is held over it, it will be felt to bulge as it transmits pressure. This is known as a cough impulse.

If the hernia cannot be coaxed back into the bowel (e.g. because of strands of fibrous scar tissue known as adhesions) it is *irreducible*. It is important to correct this surgically before it strangulates. A *strangulation* occurs when the opening through which the hernia protrudes becomes tight and constricts the circulation to the bowel. This causes symptoms of severe pain in the hernia itself, often of sudden onset (acute), or of central abdominal pain that comes and goes in waves as if the bowel is being squeezed (colicky). The pain may not be felt in the hernia itself due to the way the nerve endings connect up to the spinal cord.

Other symptoms of intestinal obstruction soon occur. These include vomiting, distension and bloating of the abdomen, noisy bowel sounds and absolute constipation. Not even wind can pass through the constricted hernia to be voided downwards. The hernia itself will feel tense and very tender. Overlying skin may become red, hot and inflamed in the later stages.

A strangulated hernia is a surgical emergency. Even if strangulation is only suspected, medical advice should be

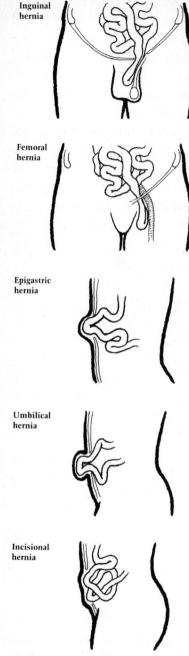

Inguinal
hernia

Femoral
hernia

Epigastric
hernia

Umbilical
hernia

Incisional
hernia

Figure 19: Hernia types. Inguinal, femoral, epigastric, umbilical and incisional hernias (in old operation scar) are the most common types.

sought without delay. If strangulation is not relieved urgently, so that blood circulation is restored, the loop of bowel will die and become gangrenous. This can cause life-threatening blood poisoning (septicaemia). The three commonest types of hernia to strangulate are, in order of frequency:

• femoral hernias
• indirect inguinal hernias
• umbilical hernias.

Congenital Inguinal Hernia

A congenital inguinal hernia is almost exclusively a male phenomenon related to the descent of the testes. Overall, 4 per cent of boys need surgical correction of a congenital inguinal hernia.

During the last few months of development, the testis travels from the abdomen into the scrotum by passing over the pubic bone. The testis passes obliquely through the lower abdominal wall into the scrotum. It carries layers of tissue with it to form a passageway known as the inguinal canal. The opening usually becomes blocked off during development, but sometimes stays open by accident. A loop of bowel can then easily trail through into the scrotum to cause a bulge. Sometimes, a congenital inguinal hernia is also associated with an undescended testis.

Congenital inguinal hernias are prone to strangulation because of the narrowness of the inguinal canal through which they have passed. They are surgically corrected, usually around the age of one year unless symptoms develop which require prompt surgery. The bowel is gently pushed back into the abdomen, the pouch of peritoneum which formed the hernia sac is tied and cut, and the area reinforced to prevent a recurrence in future years.

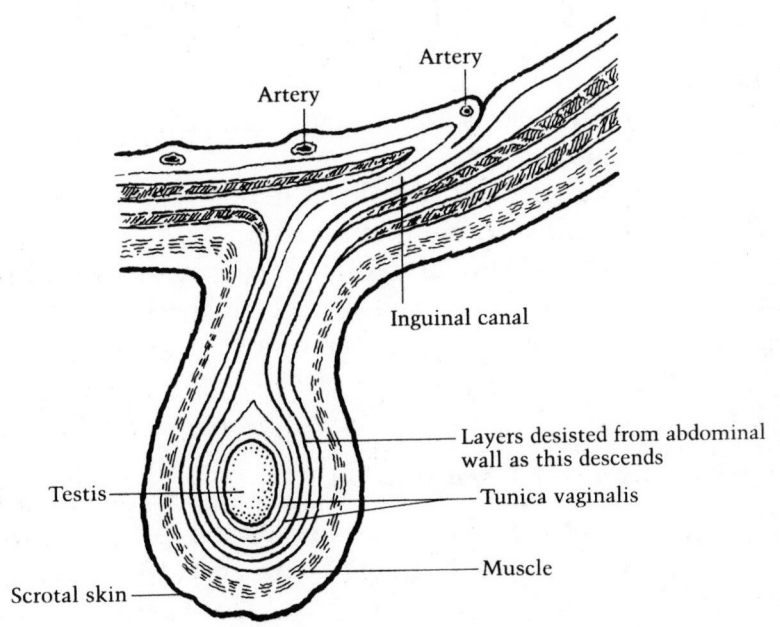

Artery

Artery

Inguinal canal

Layers desisted from abdominal wall as this descends

Tunica vaginalis

Testis

Muscle

Scrotal skin

Figure 20: A Testicle and its surrounding layers.

Acquired Inguinal Hernias

Acquired inguinal hernias are of two main types. If the bowel follows the anatomical weakness and passes through the whole inguinal canal, it is known as an indirect inguinal hernia. If the bowel pushes through the back wall of the inguinal canal to enter halfway down, it is called a direct inguinal hernia. This is because the hernia seems to protrude *directly* forwards.

An indirect inguinal hernia has to pass through two narrow openings at either end of the inguinal canal. It therefore often starts off small at the beginning of the day and gets larger once the sufferer has been up and about for a while. On lying down, it will also take time for the bowel to slither back into the abdomen (assuming the hernia is reducible). Because of the narrowness of the openings, an indirect hernia is liable to become irreducible or to strangulate.

A direct inguinal hernia, on the other hand, bulges forwards through a relatively large weakness in the abdominal wall. It therefore appears immediately on standing up and disappears as soon as the person affected lies down. A direct hernia hardly ever descends into the scrotum and, because the opening is large, strangulation is rare.

Sometimes, a direct and an indirect hernia exist in the same patient on the same side simultaneously.

Sixty per cent of inguinal hernias occur on the right-hand side, 20 per cent on the left, and 20 per cent are bilateral. They vary in size from small bulges to enormous masses stretching down to the knee.

Types of Inguinal Hernia Repair

Three quarters of inguinal repairs performed in the UK still involve an old-fashioned technique designed in 1884. It is now considered obsolete in many countries. This is Bassini's darn technique, in which loops of nylon thread are used to cobble up and repair the weakness in the abdominal wall. Only one layer of tissue is stitched through, and it breaks down in 10 per cent of cases. This is the main reason why repeat operations are so frequently needed in the UK.

Two newer and more effective operations are now available. In the Open Tension Free (or Lichtenstein) technique, a patch of polypropylene mesh is stitched in place over the rupture. This makes the repair stronger and less likely to break down than other methods. The risk of needing a recurrent operation is less than 1 per cent.

The Shouldice technique of hernia repair involves stitching through three overlapping layers of abdominal wall tissue rather than one – as in the traditional darn technique. The risk of this repair breaking down are also less than 1 per cent, and more and more British surgeons are now adopting this operative method.

There has been recent experimentation with a laparoscopic (keyhole) surgery technique in which the hernia is repaired from inside the abdominal cavity and the defect patched with a small piece of metal.

Old-fashioned trusses are belt-like contraptions designed to apply pressure over an area of weakness through which a hernia protrudes. This keeps the hernia in its place but can be cumbersome. Trusses are best for small direct inguinal hernias where the pad can be accurately placed over the area of weakness. They need to be replaced every few years as they wear out, stretch and become ineffective. They should not be used where a hernia is irreducible as this can cause pressure damage to the bowel and increase the risk of strangulation.

Hernia Repairs and Male Fertility

Recently, hernia repairs were linked with male subfertility. A study in Israel found that men who had had a previous hernia repair had a one in eight chance of a small, shrunken (atrophic) testis, compared with an incidence of less than 1 per 100 in men who had not had a hernia repair.

When semen was analysed, the quality was significantly poorer in men who had had a hernia repair, whether or not they had an atrophic testis. It is thought that testicular function is either affected by reduced blood supply (e.g. damage or scarring during the operation) or from some as yet unidentified immunological reaction. These results are being further investigated.

Recent studies in Germany found that half the 834 surgeons questioned routinely remove a testis as part of a hernia repair.

233

This is obviously unacceptable to most men unless it is medically imperative (because the testis is diseased, atrophic or otherwise abnormal).

Femoral Hernia

A femoral hernia is a protrusion of a piece of intestine or fatty tissue through a weakness at the top of the leg. This weakness occurs where there is a natural gap, wide enough to admit a little finger, where the femoral vein, artery and nerve pass from the abdominal cavity into the leg.

Femoral hernias are most common in those over the age of 50. They are more common in women as their pelvises are wider, but do occur in men. They are often bilateral (occurring on both sides). Symptoms include a lump in the groin, sometimes with pain and discomfort. They frequently strangulate causing colicky pains, distension, vomiting and constipation. Once diagnosed, a femoral hernia needs urgent surgical repair because of this high risk of strangulation.

Umbilical Hernia

Umbilical hernias are protrusions of bowel related to the belly button (umbilicus). Congenital umbilical hernias form through the gap where the umbilical cord vessels enter the abdomen during foetal life. They are usually present at birth but may not be noticed until the umbilical cord separates and heals. They rarely cause symptoms and 90 per cent disappear during the first few years of life as umbilical scar tissue contracts and thickens. Repair is not usually attempted until the child is at least two years old.

Acquired umbilical hernias are common in the obese. Those hernias that protrude through umbilical scar tissue are usually caused by conditions that raise pressure inside the abdomen and distend it. This causes the bellybutton to bulge outwards. Treatment is not necessary unless the hernia is large or giving rise to unpleasant or painful symptoms.

The normal umbilicus

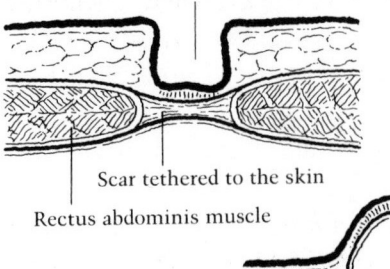

Skin dimple

Scar tethered to the skin

Rectus abdominis muscle

A congenital umbilical hernia

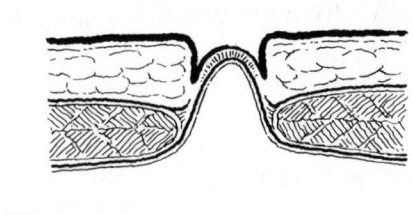

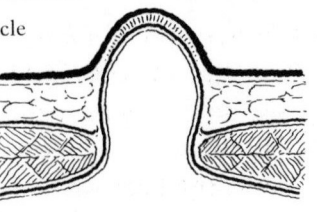

The umbilical scar fails to form or is weak. The abdominal contents bulge through the weak spot and evert the umbilicus

An acquired true umbilical hernia

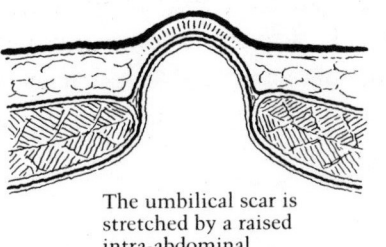

The umbilical scar is stretched by a raised intra-abdominal pressure and the umbilicus everts.

A paraumbilical hernia

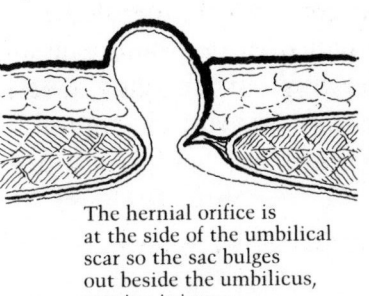

The hernial orifice is at the side of the umbilical scar so the sac bulges out beside the umbilicus, turning it into a crescent-shaped slit.

Figure 21: Umbilical hernias

Acquired para-umbilical hernias protrude through a gap to one side of the umbilical scar and convert the belly button into a crescent-shaped slit. These do need repair as they cause pain and swelling around the umbilicus and can strangulate.

Incisional Hernia

Incisional hernias form through a weakness in the scar tissue formed after a previous operation, or area of trauma. Scar tissue is inelastic and stretches easily if put under constant strain –

e.g. by lifting, chronic coughing or straining with constipation. It also becomes weaker with increasing age and if deficient in vitamin C. Complications after surgery such as wound infection or heavy bleeding also make scar tissue more likely to weaken.

Incisional hernias can be dissected and repaired surgically. If the patient is unfit for surgery, an abdominal belt (truss) is occasionally used.

Epigastric Hernia

An epigastric hernia is the protrusion of a piece of fat (and occasionally bowel) through a weakness in the mid-line between the umbilicus and the rib cage. This weakness is the natural line where the abdominal wall muscles meet. Symptoms usually include pain in the upper abdomen which often comes on after eating and is therefore frequently misdiagnosed as indigestion. Repair is a simple matter of sewing up the abdominal wall defect.

Hiatus Hernia

A hiatus hernia occurs when a section of the stomach, which usually lies in the abdominal cavity, protrudes through a gap (hiatus) in the diaphragm to enter the chest. It is more common in the overweight and in those who smoke. Occasionally, it is present from birth.

In 90 per cent of cases, the oesophagus and stomach slide upwards into the gap through which the oesophagus (gullet) passes, so that only the top end of the stomach is in the gap. This is known as a sliding hiatus hernia.

In 10 per cent of cases, part of the stomach rolls up into the gap alongside the oesophagus, so that both the oesophagus and part of the stomach are side by side in the gap. This is known as a rolling hiatus hernia.

Hiatus hernias produce two sets of symptoms: those due to

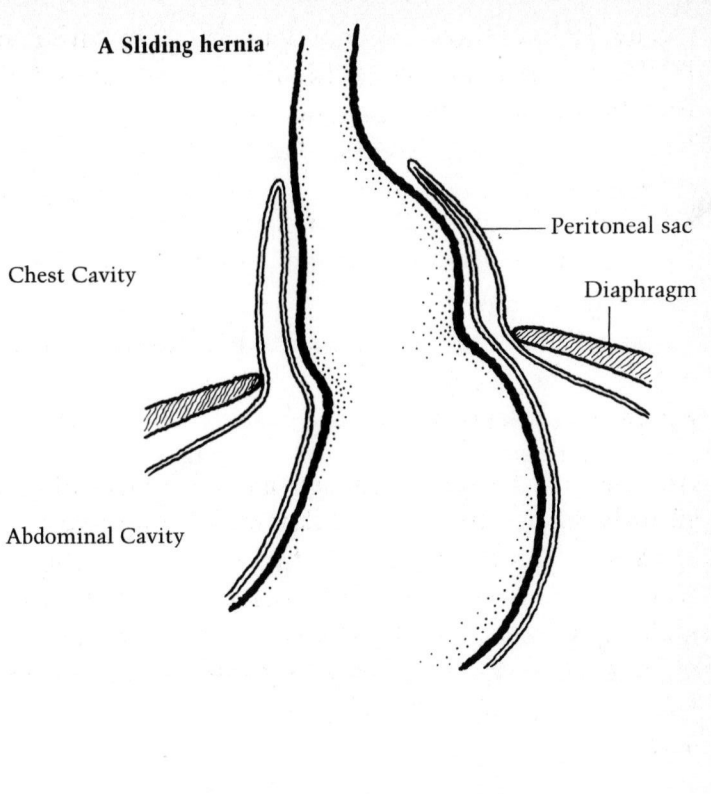

A Sliding hernia

Chest Cavity

Peritoneal sac

Diaphragm

Abdominal Cavity

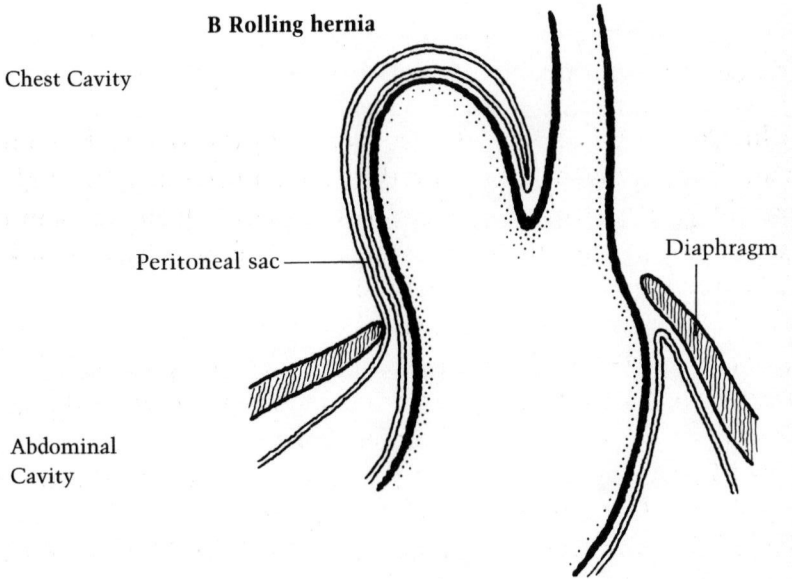

B Rolling hernia

Chest Cavity

Peritoneal sac

Diaphragm

Abdominal
Cavity

Figure 22: Hiatus hernias

the extra bulk in the chest (coughing, shortness of breath, palpitations, feelings of pressure, hiccough) and those due to disruption of the valve system between the oesophagus and stomach (acid reflux, indigestion and burning sensations which are often worse on bending over or lying down). Usually, a rolling hiatus hernia does not cause symptoms of acid regurgitation because the valve mechanism between the stomach and oesophagus is not affected.

Many people have mild hiatus hernias without symptoms, which are never diagnosed.

Hiatus hernias are investigated by passing a flexible telescope down the throat while the patient is under light sedation. This procedure is called oesophagoscopy or gastroscopy. Occasionally, a barium X-ray is also used to see whether there is reflux of stomach contents into the oesophagus.

Treatment of hiatus hernias involves losing weight, which often improves symptoms, eating little and often (rather than large meals), avoiding bending or lying down after meals, giving up smoking and raising the head of the bed slightly to prevent reflux during sleep. Some patients find they can only sleep at night if propped fully upright.

Drugs such as antacids help to reduce heartburn and protect the delicate oesophagus (gullet) from acid damage. Prokinetic drugs encourage ordered contraction of stomach and intestinal muscles and are also useful in preventing acid regurgitation.

If symptoms are severe, surgery to repair the hiatus hernia is undertaken. This is a major operation in which the protruding stomach is brought back down into the abdomen and tethered into place.

15

HAIR AND SKIN PROBLEMS

HAIR LOSS

The normal male scalp contains between 100,000 and 150,000 hairs. On average, 80–100 are naturally shed every day, to be replaced by new hairs growing through. If daily hair loss is any greater than 100 hairs per day, gradual thinning occurs.

Each hair follows its own life cycle. There is an initial growth phase lasting two to six years, followed by a resting period of around three months during which no further growth occurs. At the end of this time, the hair falls out. If a hair follicle dies, no more hair will grow and hair loss in that area will be permanent.

At any one time, 90 per cent of the hairs on your head are in the growth phase and 10 per cent are in the resting phase. Under certain conditions such as stress, thyroid disease, iron deficiency or while taking certain drugs, the life cycles of hundreds of hairs synchronize so that they all fall out at once. This causes a form of patchy baldness known as alopecia which can be difficult to treat. Left untreated, over 70 per cent of cases recover within five years. Steroid creams applied locally may help.

Other causes of localized alopecia include ringworm (a fungal infection), repeated plucking or twisting of hair and excessive traction – especially at the hairline – from pulling the hair back into a tight ponytail.

Androgenic Alopecia

Androgenic alopecia is the correct term for male pattern baldness. Hair loss occurs over the temples to cause a receding hairline, and/or from the crown (vertex) to form a circular bald patch. Androgenic alopecia affects 5 per cent of males by the age of 20 years. By the age of 70, 80 per cent of males are affected.

There is a strong hereditary component which determines at what age thinning starts and the pattern of baldness that follows. Most men inherit the same pattern of hair loss as their father had.

Male pattern baldness is androgen-dependent. Although body hair is increased by the action of testosterone, scalp hair is decreased. Blood levels of testosterone hormone are usually normal in men with a receding hairline, however, and the hair loss is probably due to the breakdown of testosterone into dihydro-testosterone *(see page 99)* within the hair follicle, which somehow switches the follicle off.

This may in part be related to diet. Men in Japan and China are less likely to develop other diseases (such as benign prostatic hyperplasia and prostate cancer) related to dihydro-testosterone levels. They are also less likely to develop androgenic baldness. It is possible that following the prostate-friendly diet discussed on page 121 may also help to reduce hair loss.

Certainly the hair is often the first part of the body to show evidence of vitamin and mineral deficiencies. For optimum hair health it is important to obtain adequate dietary supplies of vitamins C, E, and betacarotene, and the minerals manganese, zinc and copper.

Recent research suggests that male pattern baldness may be a risk factor for coronary heart disease (CHD – *see Chapter 11*). In one study, 685 men aged under 55 who were admitted to hospital with a heart attack were matched with 772 men admitted for other, non-cardiac reasons. Their degree of baldness was assessed and it was found that men with mild to moderate crown (vertex) balding were 1.3 times more likely to have a heart attack than men without crown hair loss. For men with extreme crown baldness, the relative risk rose to 3.4 times more likely, and did not seem to be related to the age at which baldness started.

It is possible that baldness is an indicator of a pattern of testosterone metabolism that in some way increases the risk of CHD. While this is only a hypothesis, it might be sensible for younger men with thinning crown hair to keep other risk factors for CHD (e.g. obesity, raised blood cholesterol, smoking, lack of exercise, high blood pressure) to a minimum. Frontal balding alone does not seem to be associated with an increased risk of a heart attack.

Several treatments are available to overcome androgen alopecia. These have varying degrees of success and varying cosmetic results.

Scalp Massage

Improved blood circulation to the scalp can encourage new hair growth. Gentle fingertip massage, plus hanging upside down for a certain amount of time per day, demonstrate varying degrees of success.

Herbalists suggest rubbing arnica cream or ointment into the scalp. Aromatherapists suggest a daily scalp massage with two or three drops of clary sage, lavender, rosemary or ylang-ylang added to 60 ml of a wheatgerm or almond oil base.

Homoeopaths recommend combining massage with taking tablets of lycopodium for androgenic baldness and premature greying, and kali carbonicum for hair loss associated with a dry, flaking scalp.

Thickening Hair Sprays

The appearance of a thicker, fuller head of hair can be obtained by spraying on a coloured agent that dries on the hair shaft and thickens it. This gives the illusion of more hair.

Minoxidil

Minoxidil is a drug originally used in its oral form to treat high blood pressure. One of the side-effects of treatment was excessive hair growth.

Minoxidil is now available as a topical solution. One ml is applied to the scalp twice per day for a minimum of four months; this appears to reduce hair loss in around 70 per cent of patients. New hair growth occurs in a third of patients but only 10 per cent produce a good cosmetic result. In others, new hair remains thin, wispy and miniaturized. The regular massage effect may contribute to the treatment's benefit.

Minoxidil is thought to work by increasing the blood flow to tiny capillaries feeding blood to the hair follicles in the scalp, thus stimulating hair growth.

If minoxidil produces an acceptable result, treatment must be continued regularly. If it is stopped the new hair growth tends to fall out again, usually within four to six months. Minoxidil treatment seems safe, with only occasional side-effects of irritation or dandruff reported. If large amounts are absorbed, low blood pressure is another possible side-effect.

Hair Follicle Relocation

This technique involves relocating healthy hair follicles from thicker areas of hair to thinning or balding areas. This is used to treat receding hair lines, balding at the temples and crowns, and generally thinning hair.

Hair Transplants

Circular plugs or strips of skin are transferred from hair-bearing parts of the scalp onto bald or thinning areas. Grafts are described as micro, mini, quartered or full size depending on the size of the plugs transferred. These are inserted into a ready-made slit or hole in the bald or thinning part of the scalp.

Punch grafting can produce an artificial, dotted appearance. At best this offers only a visual illusion of more hair, as in fact existing hair is just redistributed. Results depend on the operator's skill, the pattern of hair loss, the colour of the scalp, and the texture and colour of the hair and whether it is curly, wavy or straight. There is also the risk that grafts will not take. You are then left with an extra patch of baldness where the original plug was removed. Several operations are needed to fill in areas between previous punch grafts to produce a more natural appearance. This procedure is especially successful for frontal hair loss.

Scalp Reduction

With scalp reduction, a strip of bald skin is removed from the upper forehead before transplantation to reduce the area that needs to be grafted. This is usually done as a separate procedure, then followed by three or four sessions of hair transplantation at four-monthly intervals.

Implantation of artificial fibres

A polyethermid fibre that has the same strength, thickness and colour as human hair is available for an artificial hair transplant. Each false hair is individually inserted and anchored into the scalp under a local anaesthetic. Up to 1,500 hairs are implanted per hour.

Toupees

Excellent artificial hair pieces are now available which can disguise balding. Careful colour matching and skilful interweaving or fusion techniques with remaining hair will improve the cosmetic effect. Toupee tapes, elastic tapes and velcro can be used to keep the hairpiece in place.

DANDRUFF

Dandruff is a common form of seborrhoeic dermatitis that affects the scalp. White flakes of skin result, which are sloughed to produce an embarrassing fall-out. Some flakes are small, but sometimes large flakes form – especially if there is an associated yeast infection (*Pityrosporum ovale*) in the hair. Treatment must usually be ongoing to prevent the condition recurring.

Mild dandruff is controlled by washing the hair regularly with a medicated antidandruff shampoo.

More severe dandruff often responds to a prescription-only anti-fungal shampoo containing an agent such as ketoconazole. If this does not work, a steroid lotion (betamethasone) sometimes helps.

Alternative remedies for dandruff include using live bio (natural) yoghurt as a hair conditioner. This is left on washed hair for 15 minutes and then rinsed out. Infusions of sage, thyme, rosemary or lavender are traditional remedies used to massage the scalp.

Aromatherapists also recommend using a few drops of cypress, juniper and cedarwood in a carrier oil to rub onto the scalp and leave there for one hour before rinsing off.

SYCOSIS BARBAE (FOLLICULITIS)

Sycosis barbae is an inflammation of the beard area. It is also known as 'barber's itch'. It is caused by infection of hair follicles with the common skin bacterium *Staphylococcus aureus*. Reinfection is commonly transmitted via used razors and towels, so scrupulous hygiene is essential.

Folliculitis causes multiple small pus-filled blisters and occasional boils in any hair-bearing area of skin. It can even occur on the thighs, although the beard area is the commonest site. If not treated adequately, tiny white scars can result.

Sycosis barbae is quickly and easily improved with topical or oral antibiotics, depending on its severity. Some men have frequent recurrences which can be minimized by growing a beard instead of shaving.

Shaving Rash

If shaving causes soreness but there are not any obvious infected follicles or pustules, the cause may be an allergy to soap or shaving cream. Alternatively, some delicate skins are sensitive to a too-close shave and develop a so-called 'razor burn'. Soothing creams, lotions or ointments containing calendula, heartsease or Evening Primrose Oil often help.

ACNE

Acne is a common inflammatory skin disease due to infections of blocked hair follicles. Each hair follicle is associated with a sebaceous gland which secretes a conditioning oil (sebum) into the follicle. This normally travels along the pilosebaceous duct to reach the skin surface.

During adolescence, sebaceous glands in the skin activate under the influence of androgen hormones and excessive oil (sebum) is secreted. This produces the oily skin often associated with puberty. Skin cells rapidly divide and often produce so many cells that the opening (punctum) of a hair follicle gets blocked. This traps freshly produced sebum inside and results in the formation of the classic enlarging blackhead (comedone). The blackness is due to a dissolved skin pigment, melanin, rather than dirt as is commonly believed. These open blackheads do not usually progress to form spots. It is the closed comedone (white head) that tends to explode into a spot.

Changes in skin acid levels at puberty encourage bacterial overgrowth, particularly of a bacterium called *Propionibacterium acnes*. Another common causative bacterium is *Staphylococcus aureus* and *Pityrosporum ovale*. Bacteria become trapped in hair follicles to produce pustules (superficial microabscesses) and papules – raised pimples due to underlying deeper infection.

It is important not to pick or scratch spots and blackheads as this can make scarring worse.

In some people, inflammatory changes occur due to the bacterial overgrowth, or because of leakage of sebum into surrounding tissues. This may be due in part to an allergic reaction. White cells are attracted into the area to release potent chemicals that exacerbate the problem. Nodules, cysts and scarring result.

Acne usually affects areas rich in sebaceous glands such as the face, hairline, upper chest and upper back. In severe cases, acne may spread down the arms, lower trunk, buttock and even the upper legs.

Androgenic Acne Vulgaris

The secretion of sebum is controlled in part by androgen hormones. As puberty is a time of rapid hormonal fluctuations, acne affects 80 per cent of teenage males. Spots start to appear at around 15 years of age (two years earlier in girls) and reach maximum severity at 16–17 years. Around 1 per cent of males continue to suffer with acne into their twenties and thirties.

Hereditary factors seem to play a role. There is little scientific evidence that fatty foods, dairy products and chocolate contribute to acne, but a low-fat diet full of fresh fruit and vegetables does appear subjectively to improve skin clarity.

Acne Conglobata

This form of acne is a severe, long-term, painful disease that is also more common in males. It is characterized by the formation of large, inflammatory cysts and nodules on the face and upper trunk. These lesions heal to produce severe, disfiguring scarring.

Occupational Acne

Some males continue to suffer acne in later years due to occupational exposure to oils, tars and halogenated hydrocarbons. This is usually easily diagnosed because the site of the acne corresponds to the areas of skin exposed to the chemicals.

Drug-induced Acne

True drug-induced acne lacks blackheads (comedones) and is solely characterized by pustules. Drugs that can trigger it include corticosteroids (topical or systemic), progestogens (sometimes prescribed to males with hormone-dependent illnesses), anabolic steroids and isoniazid – a drug used to treat tuberculosis.

Cosmetic Acne

This is occasionally seen in males who use cheap, greasy lotions and creams marketed as moisturizers for men. The greases block the pilosebaceous ducts to cause blackheads, and can trigger acne. More expensive agents described as non-comedogenic will not cause this problem.

Acne Treatments

When acne is severe, prompt diagnosis and treatment are needed to prevent scarring – so never be afraid to consult your doctor if your skin starts to flare up.

Unfortunately, acne treatments need extreme patience, as often no benefits are seen for six to eight weeks after starting therapy. It is important to keep up with the treatment, however, as after two months of continued and regular use, improvements of around 20 per cent per month are common. Treatment is usually needed for at least six months.

Abrasive Agents

such as aluminium oxide, polyethylene granules in detergent or soaps help to remove excess sebum and comedones and reduce the number of bacterial colonies on the skin. They can

THE COMPLETE BOOK OF MEN'S HEALTH

irritate the eyes and skin and are of limited value. They are suitable for use in mild acne.

Washes and Soap Substitutes

are useful for cleansing the skin, removing excess grease and maintaining the correct level of skin acidity. Some are mildly antiseptic.

Benzoyl peroxide

has been available for over 20 years and is often teamed up with other agents such as antiseptics. It is applied as a cream, lotion or gel once per day and has an antibacterial effect against Propionibacterium. Studies show it can reduce the number of surface bacteria on the skin by 100 fold. Benzoyl peroxide also reduces the number and size of comedones and damps down inflammation, so that the number and size of inflammatory nodules is reduced. Studies show that it produces a 60 per cent reduction in the number of acne lesions after two months' treatment.

Side effects: 40 per cent of users notice redness and scaling of their skin after the first few days' treatment. This effect is a necessary part of benzoyl peroxide's action and generally settles down after a couple of weeks. Irritation can be reduced by decreasing the strength of solution used, by decreasing the frequency of application and by applying a non-comedogenic moisturizer. Benzoyl peroxide will bleach hair and clothes, so wear an old vest or T-shirt under your clothes after treating the back and chest.

If you are using prescribed tretinoin (see page 250), you can alternate this with benzoyl peroxide, using one in the morning and the other in the evening. Benzoyl peroxide may also be used with aqueous solutions of topical antibiotics, but not with ones in alcoholic solutions.

Azelaic Acid

is a new acne treatment applied as a cream once or twice per day for a maximum of six months. It is used to treat mild to moderate acne and has both an antibacterial and an anticomedone action. It is as effective as benzoyl peroxide, erythromycin cream or oral tetracycline.

Side-effects: mild, transient redness and irritation in 5–10 per cent of users. It is better tolerated than benzoyl peroxide or tretinoin.

Topical Antibiotics

are used in cases of mild to moderate acne that mainly affect the face. They contain either erythromycin (plus or minus zinc acetate), clindamycin or tetracycline and are applied twice daily as a solution or lotion to reduce the numbers of Propionibacterium on the skin. These antibiotics have a similar overall efficacy to benzoyl peroxide, although some Propionibacterium infections may become resistant to them.

Side effects: topical antibiotics are less irritating than benzoyl peroxide. One or two preparations fluoresce under ultraviolet light, and thus should not be worn if you are going out to a disco or anywhere you might encounter UV lights.

Systemic Antibiotics

Four oral antibiotic treatments are available: tetracycline, doxycycline, minocycline and erythromycin. Very occasionally, trimethoprim may be used. Systemic antibiotics are useful for mild to moderate acne that affects a large area such as the face, back and chest. Studies show that these antibiotics reduce the number of Propionibacterium by around 10 fold. They must be taken regularly for prolonged lengths of time, however – at least three to six months.

Minocycline has several advantages over the other antibiotics used to treat acne. It:

- can be given once per day
- can be taken with food – but not milk, which binds it
- is less likely to induce bacterial resistance
- has an anti-inflammatory action.

Side effects: long-term administration of antibiotics affects bacterial balances in the intestinal tract and can lead to oral thrush, nausea, abdominal pain or diarrhoea in around 5 per cent of patients.

In 1976, researchers found no Propionibacterium acnes resistant to antibiotics. In 1991, surveys found 38 per cent of acne patients carried bacterial strains resistant to one or more antibiotics, 26.5 per cent carried erythromycin-resistant strains, and 13 per cent carried tetracycline-resistant strains. Resistance to minocycline was less than 1 per cent. If your antibiotic (topical or systemic) no longer seems to be working, it is worth asking your doctor for a different treatment.

Tretinoin

(topical retinoic acid) is an analogue of vitamin A. A cream or gel is applied once or twice daily for a minimum of two months. Tretinoin works by stimulating the division of fibroblast cells deep within the skin. This proliferation helps push spots up and out, to such an extent that initially skin may appear worse – lumpy and inflamed – before improving dramatically. It also reduces the number of horny skin cells around the mouth of the hair follicle, allowing discharge of the comedone and restoring the free flow of sebum. Tretinoin is used when comedones, papules and pustules predominate. The majority of users show a 70 per cent response over three to six months of treatment.

Side-effects: excessive use results in thin, shiny, red skin with soreness and peeling. There may be occasional photo-irritation when the skin is exposed to ultraviolet light.

Systemic Retinoids

oral isotretinoin (also an analogue of vitamin A) is only prescribable by hospital specialists and has revolutionized the treatment of severe acne. It is reserved for patients with severe cystic or conglobate acne, and for those who have not responded to several courses of antibiotics because of bacterial resistance.

Isotretinoin is given in capsule form once or twice per day for one to four months. The dose used is dependent upon body weight and repeat courses are not normally recommended. It works by reducing bacterial numbers, preventing comedone formation, damping down inflammation and reducing sebum secretion. Within two weeks of starting treatment, sebaceous follicles have shrunk significantly in size and there is a rapid reduction in the amount of sebum secreted. The production and sloughing of skin cells within the hair follicle also decreases, which discourages blocking of pilosebaceous ducts. There is also a rapid drop in the numbers of Propionibacterium on the skin, a decline which persists after treatment is stopped. As isotretinoin does not have an antibiotic action, this effect may be related to the lessening of sebum production.

Side-effects of treatment with systemic retinoids are unfortunately common:

- facial redness in 66 per cent of patients
- conjunctivitis in 33 per cent of patients
- eczema in 30 per cent of patients
- muscle and joint aches (35 per cent)
- headaches (16 per cent)
- dry mucous membranes, cracked lips and nose bleeds
- raised blood cholesterol and triglyceride levels
- raised blood levels of some liver enzymes
- seizures, abnormal blood clotting (from low platelet count) and hearing problems (these side-effects are rare).

Despite this long list of possible complications, treatment under close hospital supervision is safe and can transform the appearance and emotional state of patients with severe acne. Monthly blood tests and supervision are necessary throughout therapy.

Cosmetic Treatment of Acne Scars

There are three types of acne scars:

1. superficial, violet coloured ice-pick scars (small pits)
2. thick, palpable scars from deeper lesions
3. ugly, excessively thickened (keloid) scars, most commonly on the shoulders, chest and back.

251

In severe cases of acne where scarring has already occurred, treatments are available to improve cosmetic appearance. These include using skin-peeling agents, skin abrasives, laser therapy and collagen injections to plump up and even out pits. Collagen injections need repeating every six months or so. Alternatively, cysts and scars may be surgically removed or injected with steroids.

ECZEMA

Eczema (dermatitis) is a common skin condition affecting millions of adult males. It is named after the Greek word for *boil*, as in severe cases inflamed skin erupts with blisters that ooze exudate or pus. Dermatitis is commonly work-related from exposure to irritant chemicals (e.g. acids, alkalis, solvents, detergents) or to allergenic substances (e.g. cement, dyes, oils, coal tar, resins, insecticides, photographic/printing chemicals, nickel, plants).

Where eczema is due to an allergy to particular foods, chemicals, detergents or metals it can be difficult to work out what you are allergic to – though skin patch-testing may help. Avoiding certain chemicals or excluding foods such as yeast or eggs until symptoms have settled down may help. The suspect item can then be reintroduced to see if symptoms return.

Eczema is often mild – consisting of a few areas of itchy, red skin usually on the hands, inside the elbows or behind the knees. In severe cases, the whole body is affected and the skin feels thickened, scaly and dry.

Itching is one of the worst symptoms of eczema and the inevitable scratching unfortunately makes the condition worse.

Nummular eczema is common in adults. This takes the form of circular, itchy scaly patches on the body that look very similar to ringworm. This is not serious and often comes and goes throughout life.

There are several ways in which you can help your eczema:

- Wear white cotton gloves under rubber gloves when handling substances such as washing-up detergents or work chemicals that may irritate your skin.
- Make sure your hands are thoroughly dry after washing – wetness will macerate eczematous skin.
- Use an unscented hand cream several times a day to act as a barrier and keep moisture in.
- Add soya or almond oil products to your bath water. Some products (e.g. Balneum Plus) also contain an anti-itch substance which soothes itchy, inflamed skin.
- Use aqueous cream instead of soap for cleansing. This does not lather but acts like cold cream to dissolve away grease and dirt.
- Apply a non-scented cream such as E45 to moisturize delicate skin on your face. A stronger cream such as Unguentum will help dryness elsewhere on your body.
- Buy 100 per cent cotton clothing to wear next to the skin and avoid perfumed products such as aftershave or deodorant.

Oil of Evening Primrose contains gammalinolenic acid – a fatty acid which feeds into metabolic pathways in your skin. This is particularly helpful for itchiness as well as dryness but needs to be taken in large doses (around 240 mg twice a day). Some men apply it directly to patches of affected skin.

Mild eczema can be melted away with a weak steroid cream such as 1 per cent hydrocortisone cream. This should be used sparingly and should never be applied to the face except under medical supervision. Excessive use of steroid creams can thin the skin, causing stretch marks or discolouration. Stronger steroid creams are sometimes necessary and are only available on prescription. Many people have found orthodox medical treatments unhelpful, but have been cured with herbs prescribed by doctors trained in Chinese medicine.

Perhaps the most useful thing you can do to help damp down severe eczema is to avoid highly stressful situations, which usually make symptoms worse.

FUNGAL SKIN INFECTIONS

Fungal skin infections are common. They include conditions such as ringworm, athlete's foot and infections of the skin folds *(see page 42)*.

Ringworm

Ringworm is the common name for a fungal skin infection that can affect any part of the body, including the feet, arms, groin, scalp, nails or trunk. It is named after the ring-shaped red, scaly lesions which slowly spread leaving a pale central area which often itches.

Ringworm is easily treated using an anti-fungal cream, lotion or ointment (e.g. clotrimazole, miconazole). If the infection is in a skin fold and has become macerated and inflamed, treatment is sometimes combined with an anti-inflammatory agent such as 1 per cent hydrocortisone (a steroid) cream. Steroid creams should not be used on the lesions without an anti-fungal agent as this can make the infection spread quite rapidly. This occasionally occurs where a patch of fungal infection has been confused with eczema *(see pages 252–3)*.

Athlete's Foot

Athlete's foot is a fungal infection that causes soreness, slitting and itching of the skin between the toes. This commonly occurs in athletes who have worn hot, sweaty training shoes for hours at a time. Fungal and yeast cells love warm, hot, moist places – sweaty feet are their dream environment.

Athlete's foot is best treated with anti-fungal creams or, preferably, a powder that helps to keep the area dry. It is important to continue treating the area for at least 10 days after all visible signs of infection have gone. The fungus burrows deep into the skin and can be reactivated if not thoroughly eradicated. If infection has spread beyond the toe cleft, for example onto the nail, oral treatments or medicated nail paints may be recommended.

Shoes should always be treated with anti-fungal sprays or powders as well, for they usually harbour the infection. If shoes smell rotten they should be thrown away and replaced.

Good foot hygiene can prevent reinfection:

- Wash your feet at least once per day, and after every sports activity. This does not mean just soaking them in the bath or standing them in the shower. The feet need to be soaped and excess skin gently pared away with tools specially designed for the job (e.g. a pumice stone, abrasive massage creams, metal parers). After washing, the feet should be dried thoroughly, particularly the spaces between the toes, using tissue or even a hairdryer.
- Clean, cotton socks should be worn every day, and your feet and shoes regularly sprayed or dusted with deodorant anti-fungal preparations. The area underneath the ends of the toenail should be regularly cleaned using a nail file. This is where dead skin builds up to harbour fungal spores.

These measures will also reduce the problem of smelly feet associated with decaying, sloughed skin and microbial infection.

16

SPORTS INJURIES

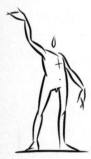

Sports injuries are common. One study found that two out of every 10 active males who regularly take part in a sport reported a recent injury. Of these, over 60 per cent were new injuries, the remainder being flare-ups of old injuries. One third of injuries occurred while playing football (soccer), a quarter were due to collisions with teammates or opponents, and a third were due to keep-fit activities such as weight training, running and aerobics. Half the injuries were muscle strains and ligament sprains. Injuries seem to be fairly evenly distributed between the arms, ankles, legs, knees and backs.

Of all the sports played, rugby is the most likely to produce an injury. The Sports Council found an average of only 20 consecutive rugby games or training sessions free of significant injury per player, compared with 76 injury-free sessions for soccer, 313 for badminton and 1,430 for keep-fit activities.

Overuse of any muscle in any sport can cause damage to the area where the muscle attaches to a bone. Part of the insertion may be torn off with a sliver of bone. This is relatively common in sports such as the discus and javelin throw.

In males, repetitive sit-ups during training cause a problem known as Gilmore's groin. Symptoms are pain high up on the inner thigh, behind the scrotum or in the inguinal region where the thigh and lower abdomen meet. The problem becomes worse on running, kicking, coughing, sneezing and after long periods of exercise. This is due to a stretching or tearing between tendons and ligaments at the base of the abdominal wall. In some cases, an inguinal hernia develops *(see page 228)*. Treatment is with surgical repair.

Most injuries are self-limiting and can be managed with rest, ice, compression and elevation, as detailed below. Rehabilitation is important to get the athlete back to his sport as quickly as possible. During periods of forced immobility it is important to maintain cardiovascular fitness through exercises which a physiotherapist can show you.

PREVENTION

Some sports injuries are preventable through proper preparation and care. The safety rules to follow are:

- Make sure you are fit enough for your chosen activity.
- Obtain proper tuition so you learn the correct techniques.
- Wear recommended clothes and footwear and use the proper protective equipment, such as knee pads, gum shields, eye protection, helmets.
- Don't eat a heavy meal less than two hours before you exercise.
- Don't drink any alcohol in the six hours prior to exercise.
- Avoid stimulant drugs. If you are on prescribed medication, check with your doctor that you can exercise safely while taking them.
- Warm up properly with a series of gentle exercises that gradually increase in intensity.
- Start off slowly.
- Stop if you feel dizzy, very short of breath, break into a cold sweat or experience any pain.
- Avoid isolated places, where it might be dangerous to be on your own.

- If out at night, make sure you are fully visible if you are anywhere near traffic.
- Cool down correctly by decreasing your exercise levels slowly rather than suddenly. This allows lactic acid in the muscles to diffuse away so it does not trigger cramping.
- Make sure your tetanus vaccination is up to date, as tetanus can occur if you are injured outdoors.

A proper warm-up routine is essential before any form of exercise. This is important because warming up will:

- improve muscle co-ordination
- literally warm your body – cold muscles easily seize
- raise your pulse rate and improve blood circulation and oxygenation of tissues
- increase your suppleness and joint mobility – to reduce the risk of sprains and strains
- allow mental preparation, concentration and relaxation, which will optimize overall performance.

EYE INJURIES

Sport is now the most common cause of eye injuries, with 42 per cent of cases needing hospital admission. Up to half of these injuries result in a permanent impairment of sight.

The sports most frequently associated with eye injury are football (soccer), squash, hockey, badminton and golf. The eye is especially vulnerable to injury in sports involving small balls and where racquets, fists and elbows flail. Of these eye injuries, 90 per cent are preventable if plastic safety glasses are used – whether or not you need visual correction of sight.

SOFT TISSUE INJURIES

The commonest sports injuries involve muscles, tendons and ligaments. Tearing these causes bleeding into surrounding tissues which triggers swelling, pain and inflammation. Immediate treatment is necessary to hasten healing, reduce stiffness and limit the amount of time you are out of action. Immediate treatment can be remembered by the mnemonic R.I.C.E.:

Rest   Ice   Compression   Elevation

Rest A sports injury should be immediately rested for 24 hours to prevent extension of the damage.

Ice packs are useful to decrease swelling of the injured area and to help numb the pain. Ice should never be applied directly to the skin as this can cause a cold burn. A thin layer of cloth or bandage should intervene. Ice should only be applied for 10 minutes at a time, then removed for a few minutes before applying it for another 10 minutes.

Compression with an elasticated bandage immediately after the injury will also help to reduce swelling. This should be applied by someone trained in bandaging techniques, as a poorly applied bandage which is too tight or too loose might do more harm than good. Signs that a bandage is too tight include pins and needles below it, pain, blueness or numbness of the flesh below (e.g. fingers or toes).

Elevation of an injured area can reduce swelling by decreasing the blood supply to the area and improving blood drainage away. If the leg is being elevated, cushions or blocks should be placed under the heel rather than under the calf.

More extensive injuries will need medical assessment, physiotherapy and treatments such as ice, heat or electrical stimulation, ultra-sonography and massage. If a tendon or ligament has been torn, surgical repair and immobilization in a plaster cast is required.

BACK PAIN

Over 70 per cent of men suffer from back pain. It is the commonest cause of time off work, with 103 million work days being lost in 1993 in the UK alone. It seems to be more and more common, with some experts blaming this on the increased popularity of aerobics and exercise routines that are ineptly followed. Even when participants are skilled, contact sports such as motor sports, alpine skiing and climbing are associated with severe injuries such as fracture or dislocation of the spine.

Weight lifters and those who play contact sports, volleyball or basketball often suffer tears in the long back extensors or the dorsal muscles due to overloading or direct trauma. Symptoms include pain and tenderness over the affected site; there may also be swelling and bruising.

Athletes with tight hamstring muscles can suffer problems with low back pain, as can those with slight discrepancies in the length of their legs. The increased lumbar curvature seen in gymnasts increases the risk of an intervertebral disc prolapse and lumbar stress fractures from the repeated landings and front and back walkovers.

Back pain can be due to:

- muscle strain, spasm or tear
- ligamentous sprain
- damage to spinal facet joints (the small joints where vertebrae slide over one another)
- prolapsed intervertebral disc
- pressure on nerve roots
- infection
- arthritis
- inflammatory disease of the spine (e.g. ankylosing spondylitis)
- vertebral fracture
- secondary cancers in the vertebral bones (e.g. from prostate cancer)

In addition to any of the above problems, pain will trigger spasm of the paravertebral muscles. This will worsen the pain and may cause a temporary sideways curvature of the spine (scoliosis).

Back pain due to a fall or accident must be thoroughly investigated to exclude the possibility of a prolapsed disc or vertebral fracture.

It is the back pain that comes on after exercise which is difficult to diagnose and which can limit activity. Only one in five cases of back pain is precisely diagnosed. The others are labelled non-specific back pain or musculoskeletal pain; 90 per cent get better without any treatment other than painkillers.

One in 10 men with backache will suffer from sciatica (pain in the buttock and down one leg into the foot) due to a prolapsed disc pressing on the sciatic nerve root where it leaves the spinal cord. Pressure on this nerve can also cause pins and needles, numbness and muscle weakness. The signs that back pain needs further urgent investigation include:

- severe pain causing immobility
- pains shooting down the leg
- difficulty with or loss of bladder control
- difficulty with or loss of bowel control
- numbness or pins and needles at the base of the spine and between the legs (saddle area)
- weakness or numbness in one or both legs.

If any of these symptoms occurs, a doctor should be contacted without delay.

Treatment of Backache

The best treatment for non-specific backache is analgesics (painkillers) and early mobilization. Bed rest should be restricted to 1–3 days, and then only if essential. If pain persists, manipulation from a physiotherapist, chiropractic or osteopath will hasten recovery.

Preventing Recurrent Backache

Many cases of backache can be prevented by:

- exercising regularly and maintaining a good level of fitness and

muscle tone
- giving up smoking – the mechanism is not known, but it seems that smoking may reduce blood supply to vertebral muscles and intervertebral discs
- lifting loads correctly by bending at the knees and hips, not from the waist. The back should be kept straight and upright as you bend.
- maintaining a good posture with the spine straight when walking – don't slouch your shoulders
- sitting square on a chair with the bottom well back and spine upright. Using the support of the arms of the chair will take some of the weight off the shoulder girdle and lower back.
- sleeping on a firm mattress and using only one pillow.

ANABOLIC STEROIDS

No section on sports injuries would be complete without a few words on the dangers of anabolic steroids. These mostly synthetic drugs are taken to increase muscle size, strength and endurance.

Anabolic steroids are nothing more than male sex hormones which have varying masculinizing and anabolic (building-up) effects. In the short term they may boost performance and sex drive, but long-term use has the exact opposite effect. They can also significantly reduce life expectation through the irreversible damage they cause to the heart and liver.

The steroids that are commonly used include: oxymetholone, oxandrolone, nandrolone, androstanolone, methandrostenolone, trenbolone, methenolone, stanozolol and various testosterone products. Many of these are designed for veterinary use. Some males practise 'stacking', in which several steroids are taken simultaneously. The long-term effects on health are frightening. Steroids can cause:

- muscle spasms
- weakening of tendons, leading to rupture
- rapid scalp hair loss

- acne
- male breast development (gynaecomastia)
- shrinkage of the testicles
- at least a 25 per cent drop in sperm count
- loss of sex drive
- impotence
- prostatitis
- benign prostatic enlargement
- prostate cancer
- undesirable changes in the levels of blood fats and cholesterol
- increased stickiness of blood
- increased pulse rate and palpitations
- fluid retention
- high blood pressure
- abnormal enlargement and weakness of heart muscle
- heart failure
- heart attack
- stroke
- liver inflammation and jaundice
- liver cancer
- constant anxiety
- mental aggressiveness (known as 'steroid rage')

and possibly:

- schizophrenia and manic depression
- depressed immunity

They are not worth it!

Part Three

NUTRITION AND LIFESTYLE

17

LIFESTYLE FACTORS

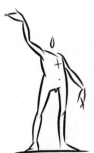

Obesity, Alcohol, Smoking, Stress

OBESITY

Over the last 15 years the number of overweight men has increased by 15 per cent in the UK. Forty-five per cent of men are now overweight and 8 per cent are clinically obese. The average male now weighs 78 kg (12 st 4 lb/172 lb) which is 4 kg (8.8 lb) heavier than in 1980.

More men are eating convenience or junk foods such as pies, chips and burgers than ever before, especially those under the age of 35. In addition, one out of every 50 males obtains a staggering 28 per cent of daily energy intake in the form of alcohol.

Fewer than half of the men aged over 24 years take regular, vigorous exercise (e.g. squash, jogging); only 20 per cent of middle-aged males take light to moderate exercise (e.g. golf, cycling, brisk walks); overall, 60 per cent of adult males take no exercise at all.

Recent research shows that being overweight during adolescence is just as important to long-term health as being overweight in later life. Males who were overweight as teenagers are more than twice as likely to suffer fatal coronary heart disease by the age of 55, regardless of their adult weight.

It is important to keep your weight within the healthy range. This is best assessed using the Body Mass Index (BMI). This is obtained by dividing your weight (in kilograms) by the square of your height (in metres):

BMI = Weight (kg) ÷ Height (m)2

This calculation produces a number that can be interpreted by the following table:

BMI	Weight Band	Male Prevalence
< 20	Underweight	
20–25	Healthy	
25–30	Overweight	37 per cent
30–40	Obese	8 per cent
>40	Morbidly Obese	0.1 per cent

This calculation is only occasionally misleading. For example, body builders with excessive muscle mass may have a BMI of up to 30 without actually being obese.

For men, a BMI of 20 – 25 is desirable as this is not associated with increased risk of premature death. If your BMI is approaching or exceeding 30 kg/m2 you should seriously consider losing weight. Your risk of premature death doubles as BMI rises from 30 to 40 kg/m2.

The table on the next page gives the weight range for males of different heights that corresponds to a BMI of 20–25. This lets you see whether or not you are in the healthy weight bracket.

Excess weight goes on when energy intake exceeds energy output over a prolonged period of time. Being fat indicates you have eaten more than you have required over the years. Various factors determine how many calories you need per day. These include your level of activity and our metabolic rate.

From the age of 27 your metabolic rate naturally slows by as much as 12 per cent over the next 20 years. You therefore need

Height		Optimum male weight range (BMI of 20–25)	
Metres	Feet	Kilograms	Stones and pounds
1.68	5'6"	56–70	8 st 12 lb–11 st (124–154 lb)
1.70	5'7"	58–72	9 st 1 lb–11 st 4 lb (127–158 lb)
1.73	5'8"	60–75	9 st 6 lb–11 st 10 lb (132–164 lb)
1.75	5'9"	61–76	9 st 9 lb–12 st (135–168 lb)
1.78	5'10"	63–79	9 st 13 lb–12 st 6 lb (139–174 lb)
1.80	5'11"	65–81	10 st 3 lb–12 st 9 lb (143–177 lb)
1.83	6'	67–83	10 st 7 lb–13 st 1 lb (147–183 lb)
1.85	6'1	69–85	10 st 11 lb–13 st 5 lb (151–187 lb)
1.88	6'2"	71–88	11 st 2 lb–13 st 12 lb (156–194 lb)
1.90	6'3"	72–90	11 st 5 lb–14 st 2 lb (159–198 lb)
1.93	6'4"	75–93	11 st 10 lb–14 st 8 lb (164–204 lb)

to eat less or exercise more as you get older to prevent a gain in weight – even if your daily intake stays the same. In practice, you tend to eat more and exercise less with increasing age, hence the dreaded middle-age spread.

Calorie Needs

The number of daily calories you need depends on your age, your current weight and your general level of activity. To find out how many calories you are likely to need per day just to maintain your weight, first work out which activity level you fall into:

Activity Level 1: Spending most of the day sitting at a desk, reading, watching TV, writing, listening to the radio. No sport

Activity Level 2: Spending most of the day driving, playing a musical instrument, general office work, pottering round the home, light laboratory work; occasional short walks

Activity Level 3: Professional and technical workers, administrative and managerial staff, sales representatives, clerical workers, teachers, lecturers; light gardening, sport once per week

Activity Level 4: Sales workers, service workers, students, transport workers, tailors, shoemakers, electrical workers, machiners, painters and decorators, roofers, window cleaners, carpenters, joiners, motor mechanics; cycling, sport twice per week

269

Activity Level 5: Equipment operators, labourers, agricultural workers, forestry workers, fishermen, heavy-duty gardeners, bricklayers, masons, construction workers; digging, shovelling, felling trees, skiing, sport three times per week

Next, find the age group you fit into on the table below and select the weight that is closest to your own. Read off along this line until you come to the column headed by your activity level. The figure in this column gives the estimated average daily energy intake needed for a man of your age, weight and activity level.

Estimated energy requirements for adult males (kcal/day)

	Physical activity level				
	1	2	3	4	5
19–29 years					
60 kg (9 st 6 lb/132 lb)	2,220	2,390	2,720	3,200	3,510
65 kg (10 st 3 lb/143 lb)	2,340	2,510	2,840	3,340	3,675
70 kg (11 st/154 lb)	2,435	2,625	2,985	3,485	3,845
75 kg (11 st 11 lb/165 lb)	2,555	2,745	3,100	3,630	4,010
80 kg (12 st 8 lb/176 lb)	2,650	2,840	3,225	3,795	4,180
30–59 years					
65 kg (10 st 3 lb/143 lb)	2,270	2,435	2,745	3,225	3,560
70 kg (11 st/154 lb)	2,340	2,510	2,840	3,345	3,680
75 kg (11 st 11 lb/165 lb)	2,435	2,600	2,960	3,460	3,820
80 kg (12 st 8 lb/176 lb)	2,510	2,700	3,055	3,580	3,940
85 kg (13 st 5 lb/187 lb)	2,580	2,770	3,150	3,700	4,060

These estimated calorie intakes are averages only. Half the men in this category are likely to need more calories than those quoted – and half will need less.

Apples Versus Pears

Using a tape measure, calculate your waist and hip measurements in centimetres. Now divide your waist measurement by your hip measurement to get a ratio:

Waist ÷ Hip = Ratio

If a man's waist/hip ratio is greater than 0.95, the body is classed as 'apple-shaped'. If the ratio is less, the body is said to be 'pear-shaped'.

Waist/hip ratios are important. Those with a central (apple) deposit of adipose tissue seem to be at greater risk of developing coronary heart disease, stroke, high blood pressure, atherosclerosis, high blood cholesterol, gallstones and diabetes than those with a more peripheral, pear-shaped distribution of fat.

The reasons for this are not fully understood, but are thought to be related to different, inherited metabolic patterns which handle dietary fats in different ways.

If you have a BMI of over 30 and are also apple-shaped, you are significantly at risk of coronary heart disease, especially if this runs in your family. Luckily, however, people who are apple-shaped seem to lose weight more easily than pear shapes, as abdominal fat is mobilized and broken down more easily than fat stored in subcutaneous (under the skin) compartments.

Exercise can also help to change your body shape. Research has shown that waist/hip ratios can be beneficially altered with an endurance exercise programme, even in the elderly. In one study, 93 healthy volunteers (aged 60–70 years) were age-matched with suitable controls. Non-smokers who had not taken aerobic exercise within the preceding two years and who were on no medication (other than aspirin) were subjected to a controlled jogging programme or were trained on rowing or bicycle ergometers for 45 minutes, three days per week for up to one year. A pulse rate of 75 per cent of maximum was aimed for.

Following this exercise programme, reductions in skin-fold thickness and body circumference were most noticeable in the waist area. This suggests that regular endurance exercise can significantly decrease the risk of diseases associated with having an apple shape by converting body structure into the healthier pear shape.

Why Excess Weight Is Bad for You

Overweight and obesity are linked with a number of diet-related diseases in men. These include:

CIRCULATORY DISORDERS

- angina
- atherosclerosis (hardening of the arteries)
- cerebro-vascular accidents (strokes)
- hypertension (high blood pressure)
- myocardial infarction (heart attack)
- peripheral vascular disease (poor circulation)
- varicose veins

METABOLIC DISORDERS

- diabetes
- hyperlipidaemia (high blood cholesterol/fats)
- gout
- haemorrhoids

GASTRO-INTESTINAL DISORDERS

- acid reflux (heartburn)
- cholelithiasis (gall stones)
- diverticular disease
- Inflammatory bowel disease
- irritable bowel syndrome

RESPIRATORY DISORDERS

- breathlessness
- hypoventilation (under-breathing)
- sleep apnoea (snoring; lack of oxygen at night)

MUSCULO-skeletal PROBLEMS

- back pain
- osteoarthritis
- joint pains

IMMUNOLOGICAL DISORDERS

- auto-immune disease
- eczema
- frequent infections

CANCERS

- bladder
- prostate gland
- stomach
- pancreas
- colon
- rectum

REPRODUCTIVE PROBLEMS

- lower sperm count
- lower libido
- subfertility

If you are overweight you need to do something about it now, not wait for a bad back or your first heart attack to galvanize you into action.

How to Lose Weight Safely

The only way to lose weight is to eat fewer calories than you burn. It is best to do this slowly, at a rate of around 0.5 – 1 kg (1 – 2 lb) weight loss per week. If you lose weight more rapidly than this two undesirable things will happen:

1. you will lose a greater percentage of lean tissue mass (muscle)
2. your metabolism will go onto 'red alert' and slow by up to 30%.

Then, as soon as you started eating more, your body fat stores would pile back on again – but not the muscle you lost. You could end up weighing more, with less of that weight composed of muscle, than before you decided to diet.

The best way to lose weight permanently is to change your eating habits, so that you eat more healthily without feeling you are actually 'on a diet', and to increase the amount of exercise you take.

Eating More Healthily

Aim to eat between 500 and 800 calories (kcal) per day less than you need to fuel your energy expenditure. Your metabolism will raid your body fat stores to find the extra fuel it needs, so you will slowly start to lose weight.

CHANGE SOME HABITS

Switch to semi-skimmed milk, low-calorie yoghurts, low-cal salad dressings, reduced fat cheese, reduced fat monounsaturated spreads and diet or low-fat versions of any foods possible.

Ideally you need to get at least half your daily calories from unrefined complex carbohydrates such as wholegrain bread, wholemeal pasta, brown rice, baked potatoes – but do not smother them in calorific sauces.

Eating carbohydrate has a direct action on the brain to make you feel fuller more quickly. It also boosts your metabolic rate so your body temperature is slightly higher – which again burns off more fat.

Healthy eating also means cutting back on the amount of saturated (animal) fat you eat. Instead of having red meat, go for lean chicken with the skin removed, and eat more fish and vegetarian meals. Grill food rather than frying; bake instead of roasting.

Do not be tempted to miss meals – always eat breakfast, lunch and dinner as eating boosts your metabolic rate and keeps it running at an optimal high. Between-meal snacks are fine as long as you stick to low-calorie yoghurt, fresh fruit or unsweetened wholegrain biscuits, and reduce the size of your main meals accordingly.

An easy guide to healthy eating is outlined below. The general rule of thumb is:

- Avoid RED foods.
- Go easy on AMBER foods.
- Eat as many GREEN foods as you like.

Red	*Amber*	*Green*
Sugar	Honey	Fresh beans
Sugary fizzy drinks	Cheese	Lettuce etc.
Sweets	Avocado	Tomatoes
Chocolate	Red Meat	Cucumber
Cakes	*Unsweetened Cereals	Carrots
Biscuits	Semi-skimmed milk	Onions
Sponge, gateaux	Diet mayonnaise	Peppers
Doughnuts	Unsweetened Juice	Lentils
Sweetened cereals	Dried Fruit	Seeds
Jam, syrup	*Wholegrain Bread	Radish
Marmalade	*Wholemeal pasta	Sweetcorn
Alcohol	*Potatoes	Beetroot
Fatty meat	*Brown Rice	Cauliflower
Full cream milk	Eggs (× 2 per week)	Mushrooms
Crisps	Unsalted Nuts	Peas
Salted nuts	Baked beans	Cabbage
Peanut butter	Bananas	Greens
Mayonnaise		Fresh fruit
Oily salad dressings		White meat
Salad cream		Fish
Butter		Prawns
Cream		Cottage cheese
Sour cream		Skimmed milk
Ice cream		Low fat yoghurt
Custard		Fresh herbs
Puddings of any sort		
Fried foods		
Bacon		
Fatty sausages		
Salami		
Paté		
Pastry		
Cream Soup		
Sauces		
Chips		

*at least half your daily energy intake should come from these sources

Exercise

Increased levels of activity burn up more calories, so losing weight should always be a combination of eating more healthily, eating low-fat foods and increasing your exercise levels.

Recreational exercise such as brisk walking, cycling, swimming or working out at a gym is especially important if you spend most of the day sitting down or standing relatively still on your feet.

Lack of exercise encourages a sluggish metabolism, weight gain, high blood pressure and high blood cholesterol levels, and inhibits the way your body handles glucose.

In comparison, regular physical exercise has positive effects on health. It curbs the appetite, boosts metabolic rate and makes you feel energized, as well as:

- improving strength, stamina and suppleness
- reducing blood cholesterol levels
- reducing high blood pressure
- improving the efficiency of your heart
- strengthening bones
- relieving depression.

Regular exercise can significantly cut the risk of a stroke in middle-aged men. A study of almost 8,000 men aged 40–59 showed that in the group of inactive males (who took no exercise at all), 3.1 per 1,000 males suffered a stroke per year. In the group who took occasional gentle exercise such as gardening, 2.3 strokes occurred per 1,000 men per year. For men who took light exercise with regular walks, the figure dropped to 1.7 per 1,000; for those who took moderate exercise, such as cycling or frequent recreation, the rate was 1.4 strokes per 1,000, and for those who regularly played sport once per week, the risk dropped to 1 per 1,000 men per year. In men who exercised intensely three times per week, the risk of a stroke fell to a mere 0.5 per 1,000 men per year.

Further studies have shown that men who exercise vigorously on a regular basis are half as likely to suffer from coronary heart disease than men who take no vigorous exercise at all.

Strength, Stamina and Suppleness

Exercise improves strength by building up muscle bulk, increases stamina by boosting muscle energy stores, and heightens suppleness by enhancing the range of movement in joints and making ligaments and tendons more flexible.

Different sports contribute to strength, stamina and suppleness in different ways:

To achieve fitness you should start off slowly and take regular exercise lasting at least 20 minutes, for a minimum of three times per week. Once you have achieved a reasonable

The health benefits of different sports

Activity	Stamina	Suppleness	Strength
Aerobics	***	***	**
Athletics	***	**	***
Badminton	**	***	**
Circuit training	***	***	***
Cricket	*	**	*
Cycling	****	**	***
Football (soccer)	***	***	***
Golf	*	**	*
Jogging	****	**	**
Karate/judo	*	**	*
Rounders (baseball)	**	*	**
Rowing	***	*	**
Skiing (downhill)	**	**	**
Skipping	***	**	**
Squash	***	***	**
Swimming (hard)	****	****	****
Tennis	**	***	**
Walking (ramble)	**	*	*
Walking (brisk/hill)	***	*	**
Weight training	*	**	****
Yoga	*	***	*

* = slight effect ** = beneficial effect
*** = very good effect **** = excellent effect

level of fitness, you should do more.

Non-weight-bearing exercises such as cycling or swimming are excellent for those with joint problems such as mild arthritis, but if you have not taken much exercise during the last six months, start off slowly, perhaps with brisk walks, or with swimming or cycling on the flat. If you are relatively unfit do not launch straight into a jogging programme and do not take up squash.

Squash is one of the most dangerous games for any man over the age of 40, with a high risk of sudden death from heart attack on court. Some cardiac specialists recommend that no man plays squash over the age of 40 years. It is a doubly dangerous game for men who are overweight or unfit.

Always start a new sport gently and work up to higher effort levels using your pulse as a guide. Make sure you warm up before exercising and cool down afterwards.

> *NB* If you suffer from any medical condition (especially a heart problem) or are on any prescribed drugs, always consult your doctor before starting an exercise programme.

Using Your Pulse Rate

Measuring your pulse rate during exercise will ensure you stay within exercise levels that are safe and most efficient for burning fat and gaining fitness. Your pulse can be most easily felt:

- on the inner wrist on the same side as your thumb (radial pulse)
- at the side of the neck, under the jaw (carotid pulse).

Find your pulse and count it after sitting quietly for around 15 minutes. The heart beats approximately 70 times per minute in the averagely fit man.

Resting pulse rate (beats per minute)	Level of fitness
50–59	Excellent (trained athletes)
60–69	Good
70–79	Fair
80 or over	Poor

Now, calculate your maximum pulse rate. This equals:

220 – Your Age (see chart below)

Activity levels need to increase your heart rate to between 60 and 80 per cent of this estimated maximum, as calculated on the chart below. This will ensure your exercise programme is improving your fitness levels without putting your heart under undue strain. At the end of a 20-minute exercise period you should end up feeling invigorated rather than exhausted. It is easiest to count your pulse over a 10-second period while exercising, so 10-second pulse ranges corresponding to your target pulse rate per minute are also given:

Exercise pulse rates to aim for

Age	Estimated max. pulse rate (220 – age)	60% max. pulse rate	80% max. pulse rate	10-second pulse range
20	200	120	160	20–27
25	195	117	156	20–26
30	190	114	152	19–25
35	185	111	148	19–25
40	180	108	144	18–24
45	175	105	140	18–23
50	170	102	136	17–23
55	165	99	132	17–22
60	160	96	128	16–21
65	155	93	124	16–21
70	150	90	120	15–20

If you are unfit, make sure your pulse stays at the lower end of the 10-second pulse training range to begin with; slowly work up to a higher pulse rate over a few weeks. If your pulse rate is higher than it should be, stop exercising and walk around slowly until your pulse rate slows. Then restart your exercise but take things less vigorously.

Take your pulse every 10 minutes during your exercise period, and again immediately after you finish.

Try taking your pulse one minute after you stop exercising,

too. The more rapidly your pulse rate falls, the fitter you are. After 10 minutes rest your heart rate should fall to below 100 beats per minute. If you are very fit your pulse will drop by up to 70 beats in one minute.

ALCOHOL

Alcohol is a drug that should be treated with respect. While a healthy intake can reduce the risk of a heart attack, excessive amounts can cause high blood pressure, lowered testosterone levels, lowered sex drive, impotence ('brewer's droop') and low sperm count. More importantly, the breakdown product of alcohol, acetaldehyde, is a cellular poison which can result in damage to liver cells, brain cells and heart muscle.

The most convenient way to monitor your alcohol intake is to measure the number of units of alcohol you drink per week, where:

> 1 unit alcohol = 100 ml (one glass) of wine
> = 50 ml (one measure) of sherry
> = 25 ml (single tot) of spirit
> = 300 ml (½ pint) of beer.

NB In the US, a unit of alcohol is called a drink

The healthy maximum alcohol intake for men is currently accepted as 21 units. Most men tend to overestimate the strength of spirits and underestimate the strength of beer. For example, a man drinking two pints of beer has consumed *four* units. A man drinking two glasses of wine and a double vodka has also consumed *four* units.

Some studies are starting to suggest that men can drink up to 30 units per week without increasing their risk of serious disease. Until these studies are verified, however, it is wise to stick to the 21-unit cut off.

Other studies show that men who regularly drink more than three pints of beer a day (six units) are at twice the risk of sudden cardiac death than those drinking moderately (one to two pints/two to four units per day).

Binge drinkers and those who drink heavily only at weekends and holidays are also more at risk of sudden death. There is no doubt that drinking more than 50 units of alcohol per week will seriously endanger your health.

The form of alcohol which seems most beneficial to health, in moderation, is red wine. The US Food and Drug Administration even allows vintners to label red wines as 'good for the health', which is quite remarkable. At least 20 studies around the world have shown that a moderate intake of alcohol (two to four units per day) reduces the risk of coronary heart disease by 40 per cent. Red wine, especially with meals, is particularly beneficial if drunk on a daily basis.

One expert has even stated that, as far as coronary heart disease goes:

A half bottle of good red wine with lunch may be a better preventative medicine than all the cholesterol guidelines combined. Alcohol is a drug that should be used regularly, but at moderate doses.

Comforting words indeed – but the alcohol content of wine may not be the sole explanation for these cardio-protective effects. Red wine, non-alcoholic red wine and red grape juice all contain many unusual antioxidants which are thought to prevent oxidation of cholesterol in the blood and discourage furring up of the arteries. They also decrease the stickiness of blood, thereby reducing the risk of a thrombosis (blood clot).

In one study of 129,000 people, the cause of death in participants who died was compared with their usual alcohol preference – wine, spirits or beer. After controlling for the number of drinks per day, wine preference was associated with a significantly lower risk of cardiovascular death (a 30 per cent reduction for men and a 40 per cent reduction for women) compared to spirit drinkers. This suggests that components other than the alcohol in wine may be involved.

Another study has also demonstrated that, in the 17

countries where dietary consumption is known, wine is the only 'foodstuff' with a significant protective effect against the risk of premature death.

Research shows that red wine contains antioxidants that are more potent than vitamin E. These include:

Procyanidins –
found in red wine at concentrations of up to 1 g/litre. These polyphenols are powerful antioxidants and free-radical scavengers.

Phytoalexins –
natural anti-fungal agents in the skins of grapes. Red wine involves macerating grape skins longer than for making white wines or champagne, and therefore has a much higher concentration.

It is thought that drinking red wine with meals reduces the harmful effects of dietary saturated fats and also causes food to be absorbed more slowly. This prolongs the protective anti-sticky effect of alcohol and antioxidants on the blood at a time when dietary saturated fats – known to increase blood stickiness – are being absorbed.

Despite these reassuring findings, it is still a fact of life that over a quarter of all hospital admissions in the West can be blamed on the effects of alcohol. The long-term intake of excessive amounts of alcohol is linked with liver damage, particularly the following four pathological conditions:

1. fatty liver degeneration
2. alcoholic hepatitis
3. liver fibrosis
4. cirrhosis.

Fatty Liver Degeneration

Alcohol is a cell toxin. In order to rid the body of this noxious substance, liver cells (hepatocytes) drop their normal housekeeping metabolic reactions and frantically work overtime to convert alcohol first into acetaldehyde (even more toxic) and then into acetate.

Even a single episode of binge drinking can change liver cell metabolism and trigger fatty degeneration. Liver cell enzymes are diverted to metabolize alcohol and, as a result, dietary fatty acids are not processed or converted into the storage substance glycogen. The liver cells then start to accumulate these unprocessed globules of fat and become abnormally swollen.

The impaired metabolic reactions inside liver cells generates large numbers of damaging free radicals. This increases the negative effects of a continued excessive alcohol intake as liver cells accumulate more and more fatty globules. The liver enlarges and takes on a yellow appearance. It starts to resemble the grossly abnormal, fatty livers of the force-fed geese used to make *foie gras*.

By this stage the liver cell/enzyme balance is completely disrupted. Enzymes that break down alcohol are present in abundance, and as these can also process certain drugs and sex steroid hormones such as testosterone, more testosterone is broken down and male sex drive and sperm counts fall too. In some males, signs of feminization, such as the development of small breasts (gynaecomastia), occur. At the same time, the liver produces reduced amounts of sugars and proteins and there is an increased need for certain vitamins and minerals. A degree of malnutrition sets in.

Even at this advanced stage of fatty degeneration, changes are reversible. Liver cells have a tremendous ability to regenerate – if 90 per cent of a normal liver is cut away, remaining cells can regrow a full-sized organ.

Alcoholic Hepatitis

In a certain proportion of cases, liver inflammation is superimposed on fatty degeneration to cause alcoholic hepatitis. This may be a hypersensitivity reaction to alcohol. Cells start to degenerate and die. Some cells accumulate a glassy-looking material, while others are totally converted into balls of fat.

283

Dead cells attract scavenger white cells (macrophages) from the blood and the patient quickly becomes ill. Fever, nausea and vomiting occur, with pain over the liver area in the upper right-hand part of the abdomen. Yellow jaundice develops as liver inflammation worsens.

Recovery is followed by the formation of liver scar tissue. This process is called hepatic fibrosis.

Alcoholic Fibrosis

A liver full of fatty degeneration will eventually start to lay down scar tissue (fibrosis) even if alcoholic hepatitis has not intervened. If fibrosis is extensive it interferes with the blood supply to the liver and can lead to back pressure on vessels trying to feed blood to the liver. These swell and varicose veins develop in the oesophagus which can bleed torrentially. Fibrosis sometimes becomes progressive and leads to cirrhosis, especially if repeat attacks of alcoholic hepatitis occur.

Cirrhosis

Alcoholic cirrhosis is a serious liver disease. It is most frequent in men over the age of 40 who have drunk excessively through-out their adult lives.

Cirrhosis develops as a result of liver cell death, fibrosis, impaired blood supply and the desperate attempt of some liver cells to regenerate new tissue. The balance between blood supply and regenerating nodules of liver is abnormal, and blood-starved cells continue to die. This triggers more fibrosis, which obliterates more blood vessels. Thus a vicious circle is set up. Islands of regenerating liver cells are separated by bands of scar tissue and the liver takes on a shrunken, knobbly appearance.

Because of inadequate blood supply, these nodules of regen-erated tissue fail to function properly. Back pressure on the blood supply from the digestive tract becomes worse and the varicose veins in the oesophagus enlarge. The spleen also becomes distended and fluid accumulates within the abdominal cavity to cause gross abdominal swelling.

Alcoholic cirrhosis eventually leads to death from haemorrhage (often of the oesophageal varices), liver failure or liver cancer. This develops in around 10 per cent of cases as a result of abnormal cell regeneration.

Abstinence from alcohol at this late stage can improve cirrhosis by removing the poison that was causing the liver cell damage. Fluid accumulation is helped by diuretic drugs, and bleeding varices can be surgically improved. In advanced cases, however, a liver transplant is the only chance of a long-term cure. Fifty per cent of men diagnosed as having cirrhosis die within five years.

Drink sensibly. Do not exceed the recommended maximum safe levels of alcohol (at present, 21 units of alcohol per week for a male, which should be spread out evenly over the seven days).

A simple screening questionnaire has been designed by drinking experts to help alert you to a possible alcohol problem:

The CAGE test

Score one point for each YES answer.

- Do you ever feel you should Cut down on your drinking?
- Are you ever Annoyed by people criticizing your drinking?
- Do you ever feel Guilty about your drinking?
- Do you ever drink first thing in the morning – i.e. have an Eye-opener?

A total of two or more points means you might have an alcohol problem – see your doctor for advice as soon as possible.

Alcohol Addiction

Another useful questionnaire helps to detect signs of alcohol addiction. This was devised in the US and is short, simple and to the point. Answer YES or NO to each of the following 10 questions and add up your scores in the columns.

Question	Yes	No
Do you feel you are a NORMAL drinker?	0	2
Do friends or relatives think you are a NORMAL drinker?	0	2
Have you ever been to Alcholics Anonymous?	5	0
Have you ever lost friends because of your drinking?	2	0
Have you been in trouble at work/school through drink?	2	0
Have you ever neglected family, work or obligations for two or more days in a row through drink?	2	0
Have you ever had the shakes (DTs), heard voices or seen things that weren't there?	5	0
Have you ever sought help about your drinking?	5	0
Have you ever been to hospital because of drinking?	5	0
Have you ever been arrested for drink driving or failed a breatalyser test?	2	0

A score of six or more points indicates you may suffer from alcohol addiction. Seek advice from your doctor straight away. You need a full physical check-up (including blood tests) to see how well your liver is coping.

SMOKING

Smoking cigarettes is one of the greatest avoidable health risks a man can face. A study involving half a million smokers has proved conclusively that the risk of premature death is nearly twice as high in smokers as in non-smokers. A form of stroke called sub-arachnoid brain haemorrhage is six times more likely in young smokers than in non-smokers, and other studies have shown that smoking-related diseases kill 40 per cent of smokers before they reach retirement. On average, non-smokers live at least six years longer than smokers. Smoking cigarettes is linked with:

CARDIOVASCULAR DISEASE

- angina and heart attack
- palpitations and irregular pulse
- increased blood clotting and thrombosis
- high blood pressure and stroke
- poor circulation, which can lead to:
  - pain in the calves on exercising
  - multi-infarct senile dementia
  - blindness
  - aortic aneurysm

LUNG DISEASE

- chronic bronchitis
- emphysema

GASTRO-INTESTINAL TRACT DISEASE

- gingivitis (inflamed gums)
- halitosis (bad breath)
- peptic ulcers

CANCERS

- mouth, lip, tongue, throat
- stomach
- pancreas
- large bowel
- penis
- bladder
- kidney
- lung

SEXUAL DYSFUNCTION

- non-rigid erections
- impotence
- subfertility

There are 300 deaths per day in the UK from smoking-related disease, and doctors can now write 'smoking' as a cause of death on death certificates.

As well as affecting his own health, a man who smokes also puts the health of his children at risk. Studies show that:

- 25 per cent of cot deaths are linked with passive smoking.
- Passive smoking causes 4,000 miscarriages per year.
- Passive smoking causes asthma, eczema and glue ear in young children.
- Men who smoke more than 20 cigarettes per day are twice as likely to father children with a hare lip (cleft palate), heart defect or abnormalities of the genital tract than men who do not smoke.
- The children of men who smoke are twice as likely to develop childhood leukaemia or lymphoma (cancer of the lymph nodes).
- The children of men who smoke are 40 per cent more likely to develop brain tumours than are the children of non-smoking fathers.
- When men smoke heavily (11 or more cigarettes per day) the relative risk of their child developing any childhood cancer is 1.7 times greater than that of a child whose father does not smoke. This effect seems to be even greater if the child is male.

Some of these increased risks occur because smoking cigarettes doubles the number of free radicals produced in the body every second. These cause significant genetic damage to the sperm.

Fathers who continue to smoke while their partner is pregnant, and after the child is born, expose their family to constituents of tobacco smoke that are passively absorbed across the placenta, and by growing babies.

Health Benefits of Quitting

The good news is that giving up smoking has immediate beneficial effects on your health:

Within 20 minutes:

- Your blood pressure and pulse fall significantly.

Within 8 hours

- Levels of poisonous carbon monoxide in your blood drop to normal.
- The oxygen level of your blood increases to normal.

Within 24 hours

- Your chance of a heart attack decreases.

Within 48 hours

- Your nerve endings start to regrow.
- Your senses of smell and taste become stronger.
- The level of clotting factors in your blood reduce to normal.

Within 72 hours

- Your lung airways relax, making it easier to breathe.
- The volume of air your lungs can hold increases.
- Lung congestion, shortness of breath and coughing decrease.
- You feel more energetic.

Within 1–3 months

- Your circulation improves.
- Erections become more rigid.
- The male sperm count increases significantly.
- Walking becomes easier.
- Lung function improves by up to a third.

Within 5 years

- Your risk of lung cancer decreases by half.
- The risk of premature wrinkling of the skin decreases.

Within 10 years

- Your risk of lung cancer reduces to normal.
- Precancerous cells in your lungs are replaced with normal cells.
- Your risk of other cancers (e.g. mouth, throat, bladder) reduces to normal.

How to Quit Smoking

Nicotine is addictive and giving up is not easy. Withdrawal symptoms – tension, aggression, depression, cravings, flushing, constipation, insomnia and lack of concentration – can make you feel you are going mad. The going is tough and, unfortunately, 80 per cent of smokers who try to give up relapse within one year. Only 35 per cent of smokers succeed in quitting before the age of 60.

One of the most difficult things to overcome is the habit of putting your hand to your mouth. If you smoke 20 cigarettes a day this is a gesture you make around 10 times per cigarette, 200 times a day, 1,400 times per week, 73,000 times per year. That's a lot of habit to kick.

Try the following Quit Plan:

- Name the day to give up and psyche yourself into the right frame of mind beforehand.
- Find someone to give up with you – it's much easier to give up with a friend or relative.
- Throw away all cigarette papers, matches, lighters, ashtrays and spare packets of fags.
- Take it one day at a time – the thought of never smoking again is daunting, so just concentrate on getting through each day.
- Keep a chart and tick off each successful cigarette-free day – plan a reward for every week of success with all the money you've saved from not smoking.
- Find something to occupy your hands to help break the hand-to-mouth habit: try making models, origami, painting or drawing – anything!
- Keep active with exercise or DIY jobs in the evening rather than

sitting in front of the television. Exercise releases a brain chemical (serotonin) that will curb your craving for nicotine.

- When you get that urge to put something in your mouth, suck on an artificial cigarette. These are available in chemist shops – alternatively make your own from celery or carrot sticks.
- If the urge for a cigarette becomes overwhelming, clean your teeth with a strongly flavoured toothpaste, then go for a brisk walk.
- Avoid situations where you used to smoke, or plan ahead to overcome them: for example, ask friends not to smoke around you; go for a brisk walk during your coffee break.
- Practise saying 'No thanks, I've given up' – and mean it.

If the short sharp approach doesn't work for you, try nicotine replacement products (gum, nasal spray or patches) to see you through. Studies show that patches can double the chance of successfully giving up smoking. These should be stuck on a hairless area of skin such as your upper arm. Patches should be changed every day and not taken off at night. It is possible to swim, bathe or shower with the patches on, but don't be tempted to smoke while you are using them. The interaction of the two forms of nicotine is dangerous and can even trigger a heart attack.

Hypnotherapy

This can work where other attempts to quit smoking have failed. In one study, hypnotherapy helped 30 per cent of patients to kick the habit – making it more effective, in fact, than any other method used to help patients stop smoking.

STRESS

Stress is a term used to describe the symptoms produced by our response to pressure. These symptoms result from high levels of circulating adrenaline hormone which are secreted in response to stressful stimuli.

A certain amount of stress is necessary to meet life's challenges. Too much is harmful, however, and is increasingly recognized as a contributory factor in disease. When we are under pressure, adrenaline puts our systems onto 'red alert':

- Blood sugar is raised to provide energy.
- The bowels empty, so we are lighter for running.
- The eye pupils dilate so we can see better.
- Pulse and blood pressure go up and we breathe deeply to increase oxygen supply to muscles.
- The circulation to some parts of the body shuts down, so that more blood can be diverted to muscles.
- The testicles are drawn up safely towards the abdomen.

In the old days, this helped cavemen survive by fighting or fleeing from dangerous animals. Nowadays we rarely fight or flee, and the effects of stress build up inside us rather than getting burned off. This can trigger a classic panic attack, with symptoms caused by overbreathing (hyperventilation) and the physiological effects of adrenaline:

Physical Effects of Stress

- sweating, flushing
- palpitations and racing pulse
- dizziness, faintness, trembling
- pins and needles, numbness
- stomach pain, peptic ulcers
- nausea, nervous diarrhoea
- insomnia, bad dreams, tiredness
- high blood pressure, headache
- stroke
- spasm of coronary arteries, angina chest pain
- heart attack
- depressed immunity, with increased susceptibility to infections and even cancer

Mental Effects of Stress

- overwhelming feelings of anxiety and panic

- inability to cope
- fear of failure
- fear of rejection
- loss of ability to concentrate
- loss of sex drive, impotence
- premature or retarded ejaculation
- reliance on alcohol, smoking, drugs
- obsessive or compulsive behaviour
- feelings of isolation from colleagues and friends
- a feeling of impending doom

Stress comes from two main sources: internal and external pressures.

Internal pressures would include forcing yourself to work long hours, lack of time off for relaxation, lack of sleep, physical unfitness, exhaustion and the effects of disrupted biorhythms (such as are caused by jet lag or working night shifts).

Other internal sources of stress include uncertainty of goals in life and having a negative self-image, which leads to constant questioning of your own self-worth. Certain personality traits lead to excessive stress due to competitive behaviour, a continual sense of urgency and an inability to slow down.

External pressures are mainly related to change. There may be changes in relationships, in the family or at work. Changes often bring feelings of frustration and of not being in control.

Most stress is self-generated, however, for although an external factor may be the stimulus, it is how you react to it that is important.

Coping with Stress

The best way to cope with stress is to adapt to it in a positive, constructive manner. Situations must be seen in perspective, problems analysed logically and plans made to resolve them. Psychologists recommend the following:

- Work out what situations and people cause you stress, and why.

293

Often only a few sources are involved and you may be able to change or adapt to them in a positive manner.

- Change those things that can be changed, then learn to accept those that cannot be altered.
- Formulate decisions in unhurried circumstances, not under deadline pressures.
- Set realistic goals – tackle big problems one step at a time.
- Expect to make mistakes. Apologize then learn from them. Don't give up when the going gets tough – this is a waste of valuable experience.
- Learn to be patient and to lose your great sense of urgency, especially when driving. For example, let pushy drivers get in front of you rather than speeding up so they cannot get in; stop at amber lights instead of racing through just-red ones.
- Talk more slowly and listen without interrupting.
- Be assertive. Say 'No' and mean it. This will help prevent you being put-upon and overloaded with tasks.
- Identify and respect your good points. Improve your shortcomings as much as possible, then accept them as part of you.
- Don't compare yourself unfavourably with others.
- Don't expect others to change before you are prepared to change yourself.

Exercise

Regular exercise such as swimming, walking, cycling or other non-competitive sport is essential in overcoming stress. Adrenaline has primed you for activity: exercising will help you use this energy and reset your stress responses to a lower level.

Relaxation

Relaxation helps to switch off the body's stress responses. One of the most successful ways of dealing with stress is to learn to relax. Set aside an hour (or four periods of 15 minutes each) every day to sit down quietly and read, or just close your eyes and rest.

Many complementary therapies can help to overcome stress and encourage relaxation. These include massage, acupuncture, flotation therapy, herbal medicine, homoeopathy, yoga, reflexology, aromatherapy, and hypnotherapy. Experiment with a few until you find one that suits you and induces relaxation.

Diet and Stress

Caffeine and nicotine mimic the body's stress response and are best avoided when you are under real pressure. Limit tea and coffee to three cups per day. Better still, switch to decaffeinated brands.

Vitamin C and the vitamin B complexes are depleted under stress as they are rapidly used up in the metabolic reactions associated with the fight-or-flight response. Vitamin B is further depleted by the metabolism of alcohol and sugary foods, often resorted to in difficult times. Vitamin B deficiency in itself leads to symptoms of anxiety and irritability, so a vicious circle is propagated. Dietary tips that will help you fight the effects of stress include:

- Eat high-fibre whole foods.
- Decrease your intake of sugar, salt and saturated fats.
- Eat little and often to prevent hypoglycaemia (low blood sugar levels), which also trigger the release of adrenaline and heighten the symptoms of stress.
- If you smoke, try to stop. In the short term smoking may seem to quell your stress, but in the long term it will magnify the harmful effects of stress on your health.
- Keep alcohol intake to within the safe maximum.
- Above all, learn to relax. Go swimming, cycling or play a non-competitive sport. Take a stroll round the park during your lunch break. Treat yourself to half an hour in a jacuzzi, or to an aromatherapy massage. Whatever you do, allow some time to yourself to relax fully.

295

Stress Busters

Herbal supplements known as adaptogens can help you cope better at times of stress. An adaptogen is a substance that strengthens, normalizes and regulates all the body's systems. It has wide-ranging, beneficial actions and boosts your immunity through several different actions rather than one specific effect. This helps you adapt to a wide variety of new or stressful situations. Research suggests that adaptogens work by increasing energy production in body cells by boosting oxygen uptake and the processing of cell wastes. This encourages cell growth and increases cell survival. Adaptogens have been shown to normalize blood sugar levels, hormone synthesis, the effects of stress and disrupted biorhythms.

Adaptogens seem to work best as energy stimulants and stress busters if fatigue is not directly due to excess physical exertion but to an underlying problem such as a poor or irregular diet, hormone imbalance, stress or excess consumption of coffee, nicotine or alcohol. When adaptogens are used together with vitamin C and the B complex vitamins, results are often improved.

GINSENG (PANAX GINSENG; P QUINQUEFOLIUM)

Chinese (or Korean) ginseng is a powerful adaptogen. White ginseng is produced from air-drying the root, while red ginseng (which is more potent and stimulating) is produced by steaming and then drying the root. The closely related American ginseng has a similar action but is said to be sweeter-tasting and to have more 'yin' (heat-reducing capacity) than Chinese ginseng.

Ginseng has been used in the Orient as a revitalizing and life-enhancing tonic for over 7,000 years. Its root contains a variety of hormone-like substances known as ginsenosides which are thought to increase production of a pituitary hormone (adrenocorticotrophic hormone – ACTH) that kick-starts the adrenal glands to improve their ability to function during times of stress. Ginseng helps the body adapt to physical or emotional stress and fatigue by improving physical and mental energy levels, stamina, strength, alertness and concentration. Research suggests that American ginseng contains more of the calming and relaxing Rb1 ginsenosides, while Korean ginseng contains more of the stimulating Rg1 ginsenosides.

Dose

Depends on grade of root. Choose a standardized product, preferably with a content of at least 5 per cent ginsenosides for American ginseng and 15 per cent ginsenosides for Korean ginseng. Start with a low dose and work up from 200 – 1,000 mg per day. Most people find their optimum dose is around 600 mg daily. In the East, ginseng is taken in a two-weeks-on, two-weeks-off cycle. It should not be taken for more than six weeks without a break.

Ginseng should not be used by men with high blood pressure or glaucoma.

It is best to avoid taking other stimulants such as caffeine-containing products and drinks while taking ginseng.

SIBERIAN GINSENG (*ELEUTHEROCOCCUS SENTICOSUS*)

Siberian ginseng is another powerful adaptogen with similar actions to Korean ginseng. It contains unique substances known as eleutherosides which help the body to adapt and cope during times of stress. Siberian ginseng is used extensively to improve stamina and strength, particularly when suffering from stress, fatigue or illness. It increases the number and activity of immune cells, and Russian research shows that those taking it regularly have 40 per cent fewer colds, 'flu and other infections, and take a third fewer days off work due to health problems than those not taking it.

Siberian ginseng is also used to counter jet lag, and has been shown to help normalize high blood pressure, raised blood sugar levels and abnormal blood clotting. It is therefore used to reduce the risk of heart disease and to maintain a healthy circulation. It is particularly popular with athletes as it can significantly improve performance and reaction times by decreasing lactic acid build-up in muscles, increasing glycogen storage by as much as 80 per cent, boosting energy levels, maximizing oxygen usage and speeding production of new red blood cells. In a study of 12 male athletes, those taking Siberian ginseng increased their total exercise duration by almost a quarter (23.3 per cent), compared with only 7.5 per cent for those taking placebo.

Dose

Siberian ginseng capsules: 1 – 2 grams per day. Occasionally up to 6 g daily is recommended. Choose a brand standardized to contain more than 1 per cent for eleutherosides.

Start with a low dose in the morning at least 20 minutes before eating. If increasing the dose, work up slowly and take two or three times per day. Take daily for two to three months, then have a month without. Most users notice a difference after just five days. Do not use (except under medical advice) if you suffer from high blood pressure, a tendency to nose bleeds, insomnia, rapid heart beat (tachycardia), high fever or congestive heart failure.

A Simple Relaxation Exercise

Find somewhere quiet and warm to lie down. This exercise is especially beneficial after a long soak in a warm bath.

Remove your shoes and loosen tight clothing, especially your belt and tie. You are going to work round your body, tensing and relaxing different muscle groups to relieve tension. Close your eyes and keep them closed throughout the relaxation exercise.

First, lift your **forearms** into the air. Bend them at the elbow and clench your **fists** hard. Concentrate only on the tension in these muscles.

Breathe in deeply and slowly. As you breathe out, start to relax and let the tension in your arms drain away. Release your clenched fists and lower your arms gently down beside you. Feel the tension flow out of them until your fingers start to tingle. Your arms may start to feel like they do not belong to you. Keep breathing gently and slowly.

Now tense your **shoulders and neck**, shrugging your shoulders up as high as you can. Feel the tension in your head,

298

shoulders, neck and chest. Hold it for a moment. Then, slowly let the tension flow away. Breathe gently and slowly as the tension flows away.

Now lift your **head** up and push it forwards. Feel the tension in your neck. Tighten all your **facial muscles**. Clench your teeth, frown and screw up your eyes. Feel the tension on your face, the tightness in your skin and jaw, the wrinkles on your brow.

Hold this tension for a few seconds then start to relax. Let go gradually, concentrating on each set of muscles as they relax. A feeling of warmth will spread across your head as the tension is released. Your head will feel heavy and very relaxed.

Continue in this way, working next on your **back** muscles (providing you do not have a back problem) by pulling your shoulders and head backwards and arching your back upwards. Hold this for a few moments before letting your weight sink comfortably down as you relax. Check your arms, head and neck are still relaxed, too.

Pull in your **abdomen** as tightly as you can. Then, as you breathe out, slowly release and feel the tension drain away. Now blow out your stomach as if tensing against a blow. Hold this tension for a few moments, then slowly relax.

Make sure tension has not crept back into parts of your body you have already relaxed. Your upper body should feel heavy, calm and relaxed.

Now, concentrate on your **legs**. Pull your **toes** up towards you and feel the tightness down the front of your legs. Push your toes away from you and feel the tightness spread up your legs. Hold this for a few moments, then lift your legs into the air, either together or one at a time. Hold for a few moments and then lower your legs until they are at rest.

Relax your thighs, buttocks, calves and feet. Let them flop under their own weight. Feel the tension flow down your legs and out through your toes. Feel your legs become heavy and relaxed. Your toes may tingle.

Your whole body should now feel very heavy and very relaxed. Breathe calmly and slowly and feel all that tension drain away.

Imagine you are lying in a warm, sunny meadow with a stream bubbling gently beside you. Relax for at least

20 minutes, checking your body for tension and repeating the tensing-and-relaxing sequence as necessary.

Sleep

Stress is a common cause of difficulty sleeping. Research shows that:

- On average, we spend one third of our life asleep.
- One third of adult males have difficulty falling asleep or staying asleep.
- Four out of 10 adult males do not get a regular good night's sleep and consequently function at impaired levels of alertness the following day.
- 27 per cent of road traffic accidents and 83 per cent of road deaths are associated with lack of sleep.
- Long-distance drivers are more likely to crash between 2 a.m. and 6 a.m., when they have been trying to stay awake for too long.
- 20 per cent of middle-aged men and 60 per cent of elderly men snore enough to disturb their own sleep.
- Over two million men in the UK suffer from insomnia.

The commonest causes of insomnia are:

- stress
- anxiety
- excess alcohol
- nicotine
- excessive intake of caffeine
- poor sleeping conditions (e.g. noise, light, cold)
- pain
- shortness of breath due to lung or heart problems
- urinary problems (e.g. prostate disease)
- depressive illness
- biorhythm disturbances (e.g. shift work, jetlag)
- increasing age
- prescribed drugs.

What Is Sleep?

Sleep is a specialized form of unconsciousness. Two different types of sleep occur:

1. Rapid Eye Movement (REM) sleep, during which the eyes are constantly on the move.
2. Slow Wave (or non-REM sleep), during which the eyes are relatively still. There are four stages of slow-wave sleep. We enter light, Stage 1 sleep first, then work through to the deepest sleep, Stage 4.

When we first fall asleep we spend around 90 minutes in slow-wave sleep, then 10 minutes in REM sleep. Throughout the night this cycle repeats itself four to six times, with more and more time being spent in the REM stage, until just before waking when we experience around an hour of REM sleep. As a result, men who only sleep five hours per night get a similar amount of slow-wave sleep as those who regularly sleep eight hours per night.

Researchers do not know for certain why we sleep, but there are lots of theories. Sleeping rests the body and allows muscles to recover from constant use during the day. It allows the metabolism to slow down and the immune system to repair damage and fight infections. The secretion of growth hormone is triggered by going to sleep, and this may stimulate repair processes.

During REM sleep we have dreams, which seems to be important in maintaining mental health.

The pineal gland in the middle of the brain is significant in synchronizing our biorhythms and controlling sleep. By reacting to light signals received from the eyes, the pineal gland secretes high levels of the hormone melatonin when it is dark. Very little is made during daylight hours. Melatonin seems to trigger sleep and may provide a natural and non-addictive cure for insomnia. Researchers have found that volunteers fall asleep within eight minutes after receiving a small dose of melatonin via a nasal spray, compared with an average of 25 minutes for people given an inactive placebo.

Another hormone, ACTH, is secreted by the brain in a large surge just before waking up to prepare us for the stresses and strains of living. Waking up, at whatever time of day or night, is potentially harmful as blood pressure and pulse rate suddenly soar. This is thought to be why men with high blood pressure or angina are more likely to have a heart attack within the first hour of waking.

Experts now believe that people with high blood pressure need to have it controlled 24 hours a day, and that patients who suffer from early morning angina might benefit from putting a GTN tablet (or spray) under their tongue a few minutes before getting out of bed. If you suffer from high blood pressure or early morning angina, have a check-up with your doctor to make sure your condition is well controlled.

How Much Sleep Do We Need?

We need less sleep as we get older. A baby needs 14–16 hours of sleep a day, a five year old about 12 hours. Young adults sleep for an average of 7.5 hours per night, and 95 per cent of the population get between 5.5 and 9.5 hours every night. Some people seem to thrive on only a few hours each night, while others need much more.

The elderly need the least sleep of all – often as little as five hours – but often snooze during the day as well. The elderly naturally take longer to fall asleep, suffer from more night-time waking and tend to wake earlier in the morning. You must expect to sleep less as you get older. Make good use of the extra hours in the day rather than taking sleeping tablets to induce an artificial sleep you do not need.

TIPS TO HELP YOU HAVE GOOD NIGHT'S SLEEP

1. Try to go to bed at a regular time each night and get up at the same time each morning.
2. Make sure your bed is comfortable, the room warm, dark and quiet.
3. Get into a bedtime routine – brushing teeth, bathing, setting

the alarm – to 'set the mood' for sleep.

4. Avoid things that interfere with sleep (e.g. caffeine, nicotine, alcohol, rich and heavy foods) – especially in the evenings.

5. Don't drink too much fluid in the evening – a full bladder is guaranteed to disturb your rest.

6. If you can't sleep, don't toss and turn. Get up and read or watch television for half an hour. When you feel sleepy, go back and try again. If sleep does not come within 15 minutes, get up and repeat this process.

7. Avoid napping during the day if you have difficulty sleeping at night.

8. Regular exercise every day will help. Active people sleep more easily – but don't take strenuous exercise late in the evening. Gentle exercise such as walking an hour or two before bedtime is fine.

Alternative therapies for encouraging a good night's sleep include a course of acupuncture, reflexology, flotation therapy or massage.

Many soothing herbal infusions (tisanes, teas) containing sleep-inducing herbs such as valerian, hops and passionflower are widely available. Homoeopathic remedies including coffea, pulsatilla and rhus tox can be helpful (taken before midnight). After midnight, try arsenicum, nux vomica or silicea instead. Audio tapes that contain soothing, lulling sounds are also on sale.

Sleep Apnoea Syndrome

Snoring is now known to be detrimental to health. It is linked with the sleep apnoea syndrome and most commonly afflicts middle-aged, overweight males (85 per cent of sufferers are male, with at least half being clinically obese). Early estimates suggested that 1 per cent of men aged 30 to 50 were affected, but the latest research suggests the figure is at least five times higher than this.

Apnoea literally means *without breathing*. Sufferers temporarily stop breathing for 10 seconds or longer while asleep due to partial obstruction of the upper airways.

The commonest cause of airway obstruction is over-relaxation of airway muscles. These sag and the throat partially collapses or the tongue falls backwards. Other causes of airway obstruction are enlarged tonsils, adenoids, an enlarged thyroid gland or excessive layers of fat around the neck. In all cases the blocked airway results in loud snoring. It is only when complete obstruction occurs that breathing stops. Failure to breathe reduces the oxygen supply to the lungs and causes a build-up of carbon dioxide in the blood.

The combination of oxygen starvation and carbon dioxide build-up triggers the brain to restart the breathing process. As the airway is jerked open, a gasp occurs and the sufferer may briefly wake up. In extreme cases this happens a thousand times per night – resulting in disturbed sleep and daytime symptoms of drowsiness.

Apnoea gets increasingly common with advancing age and is made worse by drinking alcohol. If the problem becomes severe, high blood pressure, heart failure and even a heart attack or stroke can result. Sleep apnoea may also be linked with an increased loss of brain cells, resulting in early senility.

Men suffering from sleep apnoea may notice daytime symptoms of:

- headaches soon after waking
- waking up feeling drunk despite having had no alcohol
- waking up with a frightening sensation of choking or fighting for air
- excessive sleepiness or falling asleep
- lack of concentration
- poor memory
- difficulty finishing sentences
- constant yawning
- deteriorating driving skills
- lowered sex drive.

If you suffer from any of these symptoms, consult your doctor for advice, especially if you have been told you snore.

A diagnosis of sleep apnoea is usually made by monitoring

patients in a special sleep laboratory. Brain wave tracings, muscle tracings and observation of the eyes, breathing patterns and blood oxygen concentrations are recorded along with breathing patterns and movements of the diaphragm. A diagnosis of sleep apnoea is made if there are more than 15 episodes of apnoea or diminished breaths per hour of sleep.

Ninety-five per cent of patients are treated successfully by a system known as continuous positive airway pressure (CPAP) in which air is forced into the airway through a mask worn tightly over the nose.

The latest procedure involves laser treatment used to make an inch-long burn down the middle of the soft palate. As this burn heals, scar tissue forms which stiffens and splints the palate, stopping it from collapsing and vibrating.

More extensive surgery may be required, such as removing and shortening the soft palate. In extreme cases, an artificial opening (tracheostomy) is made in the windpipe (trachea) at the front of the neck to allow assisted ventilation at night.

No drugs are yet available to treat sleep apnoea, but there are several things you can do to minimize the symptoms:

- Lose any excess weight.
- Avoid alcohol and sleeping tablets as both drugs interfere with the breathing mechanism and will prolong periods of apnoea.
- Make sure you get plenty of sleep – go to bed as early as possible.
- Wedge yourself onto your side with a pillow or traditional bolster so you cannot turn onto your back (lying on your back makes the collapse of the airway more likely).
- Sew a pouch containing a cork or a walnut into the back of your pyjamas. This prevents you lying on your back.
- Raise the head of your bed up on four-inch blocks to lessen the effects of gravity on your tongue.
- Special clips designed to dilate the nostrils can be bought (e.g. Nozovent) but these take time to get used to. They can also fall out during sleep.
- Special pillows that hold the head in the correct position during sleep (e.g. *Snorestop*) are available.

Depression

Difficulty sleeping is one of the important symptoms of biological depression. This occurs when the levels of chemical transmitters in the brain are made in abnormal amounts. Levels of one transmitter, serotonin, fall significantly and there are changes in brain levels of other chemicals such as dopamine.

The most common age for depressive illness to strike in men is 45–65 years, but unfortunately over 50 per cent of cases remain undiagnosed and untreated.

As well as feeling low and depressed, other signs of a biological depression include:

- altered appetite (usually a complete loss of appetite)
- weight loss
- difficulty getting to sleep
- early morning waking – typically between 2 and 4 a.m.
- loss of sex drive
- slowing down mentally and physically
- loss of interest in your surroundings
- bursting into tears
- feeling unable to cope
- feeling unworthy
- feeling life isn't worth living.

Depression is a serious problem that needs urgent medical intervention. Treatment usually involves counselling and antidepressive drugs which are effective if administered in an adequate dose for a sufficient period of time. Unfortunately, almost four out of every five people believe, wrongly, that antidepressants are addictive. They are not.

If you suffer from any of the symptoms of biological depression it is important to consult your doctor straightaway – especially if you live alone and have no one to keep an eye on you.

18

SPORTS NUTRITION

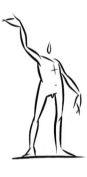

Sportspeople and athletes need to take special care with their diet. To perform at optimal levels, you must obtain adequate amounts of vitamins, minerals, certain amino acids and essential fatty acids from your diet. The harder you train, the more nutrients you need to:

- maintain red blood cell status so enough oxygen is supplied during exercise
- maintain muscle bulk and optimize contractile power
- keep metabolic reactions ticking over at a high rate.

Shortage of even a single nutrient can cause a metabolic imbalance that might impair your performance.

While you need these substances in adequate amounts, it is just as important not to overdose. Some vitamins and minerals are toxic at only 5–10 times their recommended intake (e.g. vitamin A, selenium, chromium).

It is also important to obtain the nutrients in the right balance. Too much of one vitamin can interfere with the metabolism of another. Excess zinc, for example, disrupts iron metabolism; excess iron upsets the way the body handles copper.

Too little of one nutrient can also render adequate supplies of another useless; for example, iron is no use if folic acid intakes are low – both are needed to make the blood-oxygen-carrying pigment, haemoglobin.

Everyone differs in exact nutrient needs, depending on his or her inherited metabolic traits, lifestyle and levels of exercise.

The following information is a general overview of metabolism and sports nutrition. A serious athlete will need his or her nutrient intake individually assessed and any supplements prescribed by a sports nutritionist.

BODY COMPOSITION OF AN AVERAGE YOUNG ADULT MALE

- Water: 60 per cent body weight
- Protein: 18 per cent body weight (50 per cent dry body weight)
- Fat: 15 per cent body weight
- Minerals: 6 per cent body weight
- Glycogen stores: 1 per cent body weight
  - 2,500 calories (kcal) energy stored as carbohydrate
  - 112,000 kcal (80 per cent of energy reserves) stored as fat
  - Remaining fuel is stored as protein (e.g. muscle).

THE METABOLISM

The word *metabolism* literally means *change*. It describes all the chemical and energy transformations that occur in the body, including those that convert food into energy stores and their utilization during exercise.

Ultimately, all building blocks essential for our metabolism are derived from dietary sources. We are literally what we eat.

Our body is a giant chemical reactor that oxidizes food in a complex, slow, multi-step process that liberates energy in small, usable parcels.

Enzymes (complex molecules consisting of proteins, minerals

and vitamins) are essential for controlling these metabolic reactions. They act as catalysts to trigger chemical interactions which would otherwise not occur, or would only happen slowly in their absence.

During digestion, dietary proteins are broken down into smaller units called amino acids, fats to fatty acids and carbohydrates to glucose.

These smaller units are then oxidized (combined with oxygen) to release carbon dioxide, water and energy. Some are recombined to make new complex proteins (e.g. enzymes), carbohydrates (e.g. glycogen) and fats (e.g. cholesterol) that are needed for the smooth functioning of the body. Others are stored in the form of energy-rich molecules containing phosphates such as adenosine triphosphate (ATP).

Under normal circumstances, when food is plentiful, 40 per cent of dietary energy is stored as chemical energy and used to fuel exercise and metabolism. The remaining 60 per cent is dissipated as heat.

The Metabolic Rate

The speed at which the metabolism ticks over (amount of energy liberated per unit of time) is known as the metabolic rate. This varies from person to person, from day to day and even from hour to hour. It is regulated by the nervous system and the chemical messengers known as hormones.

The metabolic rate can be estimated by measuring the amount of oxygen consumed. This is a relatively simple scientific task as oxygen is not stored in the body and consumption usually keeps pace with immediate metabolic needs.

Approximately 4.82 kcal of energy are liberated for every litre of oxygen consumed. More accurate measurements require information about the food source (protein, carbohydrate or fat) being oxidized. This is obtained by analysing the amounts of carbon dioxide and nitrogenous waste substances excreted.

Studies show that the metabolic rate is influenced by a number of factors including:

- muscular exertion (exercise)
- metabolic effects (Specific Dynamic Action) of recently ingested food
- high or low environmental temperature
- body temperature
- age
- height
- weight and surface area
- whether male or female
- emotional state
- circulating thyroid and adrenaline hormone levels
- the time of day or night
- drugs.

The most important factor is exercise. This raises the metabolic rate both during exercise and for a significant amount of time afterwards.

Muscles

Muscles are essentially processors that convert chemical energy into mechanical energy. They are the biggest contributor to the basal metabolic rate.

During exercise, blood vessels within the muscles dilate and blood flow is significantly increased to bring in the additional oxygen needed to oxidize fuel stores and release energy. This accounts for the rapid 'pumping up' effect observed during a good workout.

Mitochondria

The energy-producing reactions that occur within muscle cells take place in tiny units called mitochondria.

These are the cellular equivalent of rechargeable batteries. They are thought to have evolved many millennia ago in the primordial soup from a symbiotic species of bacteria that entered primitive one-celled organisms and set up home.

Mitochondria possess their own DNA, separate from that present in the cell nucleus, which codes for proteins and enzymes needed during energy processing.

The shape, size and DNA-makeup of the mitochondria present in your cells are identical to those of your mother. They are passed down from generation to generation within the cytoplasm of the egg from which you developed.

Interestingly, a sustained exercise programme can increase both the number and size of mitochondria within each muscle cell. This increases potential energy production and raises the basal metabolic rate.

Energy Storage Compounds

The body can easily convert protein to carbohydrate (glucose) for instant energy but lacks the enzymes and metabolic pathways needed to convert fat into glucose.

Fat stores have to be mobilized and broken down into fatty acids before they can be oxidized and used as a muscle energy source. This takes time; in an emergency situation the body resorts to burning extra protein as this is easier.

In addition, the body finds it difficult to mobilize the energy from fat molecules without a plentiful supply of dietary carbohydrate.

To use a common analogy, if excess fat stores are the logs to be burned in the fire of our metabolism, we need carbohydrate kindling to get the flames going.

Small amounts of dietary glucose significantly counteract the breakdown of muscle protein as an emergency energy source. This is called the protein-sparing effect of glucose. It is therefore essential to obtain carbohydrates before and during strenuous periods of exercise *(see page 321)*.

Muscle Fuel Sources

Resting muscles prefer to use fatty acids as fuel. During exercise, muscle energy needs increase and these are initially met by taking up additional glucose from the bloodstream and through breaking down carbohydrate stores (glycogen) within the muscle itself.

Glycogen is a storage form of glucose. It is present in most body tissues but is mainly concentrated in the muscles and liver.

Muscle glycogen stores are expandable. A male with a sedentary lifestyle will have around 1 g of glycogen per 100 g of muscle. A trained athlete may have as much as 4 g of glycogen per 100 g of muscle weight.

Muscles with a plentiful supply of glycogen are able to exercise longer without tiring. In turn, this increases muscle bulk and increases the amount of glycogen you can store.

After exercise, the muscle glycogen stores are replenished either from carbohydrate in the diet or by breaking down protein from lean tissues if food supplies are scarce.

Fatty acids, glycogen and glucose do not fuel muscle contraction directly. The mitochondria get the energy for this from the organic molecule adenosine triphosphate (ATP).

When the molecular bonds in ATP are broken down by enzyme reactions, energy is released to fuel muscle contraction and a molecule called ADP (adenosine diphosphate) is formed.

Usually, ADP is immediately converted back into the energy store ATP to provide muscle cells with fresh energy stores for the next contraction. It is for this chemical conversion that oxygen plus fatty acids or glucose are needed. Exercise is then said to be **aerobic**.

If exercise is so strenuous that oxygen is used up more rapidly than it can be brought in by the blood, or so that glucose stores run out, ATP – the muscles' energy source – rapidly depletes. Muscles then tire and lose the ability to contract any further.

A back-up molecule (phosphorylcreatine) is present in small amounts and can be used as a rich source of energy when oxygen availability is compromised. This molecule can be broken down to provide energy for the reformation of ATP from ADP without the need of oxygen. Exercise is then said to be **anaerobic**.

We cannot exercise anaerobically for long, as a waste product of metabolism, lactic acid, builds up within the muscle. As conditions become more and more acidic, muscles rapidly tire and painful cramping results.

Anaerobic metabolism in muscles is useful for providing an additional 'spurt' of strength in times of danger, stress or when quick responses are required. For example:

- in a 100-m sprint taking 10 seconds, 85 per cent of energy consumed is formed anaerobically because of the sudden increase in oxygen required.
- In a 3-km race taking 10 minutes, 20 per cent of energy is formed anaerobically. A more sustained effort is required, which the bloodstream can just keep primed with a constant supply of oxygen.
- In a slower race occurring at a more constant speed (e.g. a long-distance race lasting 60 minutes) only 5 per cent of energy would be derived anaerobically. A raised but constant oxygen demand can be met by the blood supply to the tissues.

The Oxygen Debt

Usually, the increased amount of oxygen consumed by muscles is proportionate to the amount of energy expended (i.e. 4.82 kcal energy per litre of oxygen) and all energy needs are met by aerobic processes.

When muscle exertion is great (e.g. the 100-metre sprint) and anaerobic reactions kick in to provide the emergency, self-limiting supply of energy, additional oxygen is still needed afterwards to:

- remove the build-up lactic acid
- replenish the stores of energy-rich molecules used in aerobic metabolism (ATP)

313

- replenish the emergency stores of phosphorylcreatine molecules.

The amount of extra oxygen needed is proportionate to the oxygen deficiency encountered during the period of intense exercise. An **oxygen debt** has been incurred.

Experimental measurements show that by forming an oxygen debt which can be repaid later, the human body is capable of *six times* the exertion that would have been possible without this mechanism.

There is a limit to the oxygen debt we can build up, however. Violent exertion is possible only for short periods of time, though with less strenuous forms of exercise, the debt can be incurred over longer periods.

Athletes in the peak of condition can increase the oxygen supply to their muscles much more than those who are less fit. They have:

- a larger muscle bulk
- more glycogen stores with which they can replenish ATP from ADP
- a larger number of mitochondria that are bigger and contain many more metabolic enzymes and ATP molecules
- a better network of blood vessels within the muscles bringing in blood and oxygen
- a more efficient respiratory and cardiovascular system.

Fit males can therefore exert themselves more strenuously without a build-up of lactic acid in their tissues. They will incur a much smaller oxygen debt for a given amount of exertion than would someone who was unfit.

In order for the metabolism to work efficiently, an optimum amount of nutrients are required. These include water, carbohydrates, vitamins (*see* Chapter 19), minerals (*see* Chapter 20) and co-enzymes.

WATER

We don't usually think of water as a dietary nutrient, yet it is one of the most important substances an athlete needs.

The body is made up of 60 per cent water. A third of this is outside the cells (extracellular) and two thirds inside body cells (intracellular).

During an average inactive day in temperate climates we lose around 2.4 litres through our lungs, skin and kidneys. In a hot climate, or if partaking in strenuous exercise, it is easy to lose twice this amount.

Athletes undergoing a rigorous training programme will lose over 9.6 litres per day, which needs constant replenishing. If a muscle is dehydrated by just 3 per cent it loses as much as 10 per cent contractile strength, which will reduce your speed. Your performance literally dries up.

Intensive exercise speeds up the metabolic activity within mitochondria and increases the heat output of muscles to over 20 times their resting rate. As you start to overheat, several mechanisms are activated to help cool you down.

Water is lost through the skin (sweat) to cool you by dissipating heat energy through evaporation. Peripheral vessels dilate and blood is shunted away from the intestines and muscles towards the skin. This is so that heat can pass from the blood to assist the process of sweat evaporation.

Even with constant fluid replenishment and a cool environment, heavy exercise can increase core body temperature to as much as 39.4°C (103°F) within 15 minutes (around 37°C/ 98.6°F is normal).

If air humidity is high, so sweat cannot easily evaporate away, overheating occurs even faster.

Adequate supplies of water are essential. If you become dehydrated, your body temperature will rise even further.

If body temperature goes over 40°C (104°F) your metabolism becomes inefficient and your athletic performance will rapidly fall off. More blood is pumped to your skin and away from your muscles and heart, which therefore receive less oxygen. Without oxygen, your muscles shift into burning fuel anaerobically, and more heat is generated.

Signs that you are starting to overheat include feelings of radiant heat in the face, a throbbing in the temples and feelings of coldness over the chest.

Always aim to keep your core body temperature below 40°C (104°F) during exercise. This is important when environmental temperature and humidity is high. To help maintain a safe body temperature:

- Drink plenty of water.
- Drink water that is as cold as you can stand it.
- Expose as much skin as possible to maximize sweat evaporation.
- Wear lightweight clothing.
- Wear light-coloured clothing.
- Avoid exercising in the sun. Stick to the shade as much as possible.

Preloading with Water Before Exercise

If you are training seriously for a particular endurance event such as a marathon, you can improve your body hydration beforehand by:

- eating lots of carbohydrates during the week prior to the event (see page 320). Carbohydrates are stored in the body as glycogen, which mops up water like a sponge. Each gram of glycogen is associated with 2.7 g of water. An athlete can store at least an extra litre of water this way.
- Drink extra water during the 48 hours before the event. Starting four hours beforehand, drink 200 ml of water every 15 minutes until half an hour before. Then drink nothing in the final half hour to ensure all the fluid is absorbed and your stomach is empty.

You will need to empty your bladder just before the event, but once you start exercising heavily your urine output will fall drastically. Anti-diuretic hormone is secreted by the brain to switch off fluid loss through the kidneys so that water is conserved. You will not have to worry about being caught short during the event.

Everyone has a different capacity to store water so it is worth trying this waterload regime during training to ensure it suits you.

Drinking During the Event

During the event itself it is also important to drink as much as you can. Sweat loss can be as high as 180–240 ml per mile in a marathon, which can lead to severe dehydration. This will cut your performance drastically as well as harming your health.

Even if you are water-loaded before the event, you need to drink as much cold fluid as possible during longer events. When water intake matches sweat loss, temperature rises the least and athletic performance is maximized. You will put in better times, recover faster and feel better during and after the event.

It is important to sip the water, however, not gulp it down. If you gulp you will swallow air which will bloat your stomach, reduce absorption and perhaps even trigger cramps.

Water taken before and during the event should be either plain water or contain only low quantities of sugar (hypotonic – see below). Carbonation or water containing more than 7 per cent sugar solutions will slow absorption down.

Fluid Intake After the Event

After a tough endurance event you will be dehydrated, even if you were preloaded with water and maintained a good intake throughout the event.

Although salts are dissolved in sweat and urine, you will have lost much more water than salts. You are therefore overloaded with electrolytes (sodium, potassium, etc.) and ideally need to take in plain water to correct the imbalance. Hypotonic solutions containing low amounts of glucose should be reserved until you have drunk at least a pint of plain, bottled (pure) and preferably distilled water.

Sports drinks are specially designed to replace fluid loss (after the plain water intake) as well as providing an instant energy boost to replenish those ATP molecules.

There are many brands available, which come in three main types:

1. **Hypotonic Drinks** which are less concentrated than body fluids.

These contain 2 to 3 g of carbohydrate per 100 ml.

2. **Isotonic Drinks** containing the same concentration of salts as body fluids plus 6 to 7 g of carbohydrate per 100 ml.

3. **Carbohydrate or Energy Drinks** which contain high quantities of sugars (10 to 20 g per 100 ml).

CARBOHYDRATE

The World Health Organization recommend that we obtain at least 50–60 per cent of our dietary energy from unrefined complex carbohydrates. If anything, the figure for athletes should be even higher. Carbohydrate is the most important fuel for athletes. It provides 4 kcal (energy) per gram and supplies muscles with energy twice as fast as dietary fat, which the body takes a long time to process and use. Carbohydrate is also the only fuel muscles can use during anaerobic exercise.

The basis of optimum sports nutrition is therefore carbohydrate. If the body is forced to burn fats instead, an athlete's performance will drop off.

What Are Carbohydrates?

Carbohydrates are molecules made up of carbon, hydrogen and oxygen atoms.

Monosaccharides are the simplest carbohydrates and consist of a single sugar molecule – a saccharide. The most important monosaccharide is glucose.

Disaccharides consist of two saccharide molecules linked together. The best known example is sucrose – ordinary table sugar – consisting of a glucose molecule linked to a fructose molecule.

Polysaccharides are long chains of saccharides linked together, of which the most important is starch. Polysaccharides are also known as complex carbohydrates (while sugars are simple carbohydrates). Complex carbohydrates are found in cereals, root vegetables and fruits.

Some carbohydrates cannot be digested by humans – we lack the enzymes necessary to break down their chemical bonds. These 'unavailable' carbohydrates (e.g. cellulose) pass through our bowels virtually unchanged and make up the bulk of dietary fibre – also known as roughage.

How Our Body Uses Carbohydrate

The simple sugars (monosaccharides) are absorbed into the bloodstream unchanged. The body can use monosaccharides as instant energy after processing them by adding a high energy phosphate bond (phosphorylation).

The disaccharides and starches must be broken down into monosaccharides before the body can use them as an energy source. This process starts in the mouth, with salivary enzymes, and continues in the stomach and upper intestine.

Table sugar (sucrose) is broken down relatively easily and the monosaccharides that are released quickly increase blood sugar levels.

Starch digestion takes longer and causes a steady stream of sugars to enter the blood. Eating complex carbohydrates therefore provides a constant infusion of sugar energy into the bloodstream.

Once carbohydrates are broken down into their constituent monosaccharides (mostly glucose), they are absorbed through the digestinal tract wall into the blood for distribution to the tissues.

Some sugars, such as galactose and fructose, cannot be metabolized directly by the cells and are converted into glucose in the liver before they are used as a fuel.

Blood sugar levels are controlled by two pancreatic hormones, insulin and glucagon, and also by the liver's glycogen stores, which act as a sugar buffer. When blood glucose levels are high the liver synthesizes storage glycogen. When blood sugar levels are low, glycogen is broken down and glucose molecules released into the circulation.

The Carbohydrate High

Carbohydrate triggers the release of a chemical in a part of the brain known as the hypothalamus. This chemical, serotonin, is a neurotransmitter. It relays messages across important nerve connections (synapses) in the brain. One of the functions of serotonin is to influence appetite and food selection. It regulates satiety (that feeling of being replete) and therefore controls how much we eat. Carbohydrate, the only food source that stimulates serotonin release, therefore makes you feel fuller more quickly, and for longer, than any other dietary source of energy. Serotonin also triggers feelings of euphoria. In combination with other brain chemicals released during exercise (e.g. heroin-like endorphins) this alters an athlete's perception of fatigue and improves his or her motivation to keep going. This is especially important during long, endurance events.

Glycogen-Loading

Studies with endurance athletes show that the level of glycogen within the muscles before exercise starts is directly correlated with performance. The higher your muscle glycogen stores, the longer you can continue at your maximum pace. For long endurance events it is therefore important to ensure your muscles are loaded with glycogen before the event. This is only true of longer events – such as those that will last more than two hours. For shorter events glycogen-loading would only slow you down as you are not exercising enough to gain benefit from the additional weight (glycogen plus its associated water stores) you have to carry.

Muscle glycogen stores are optimized by an intake of around 650 g carbohydrate per day. This varies from athlete to athlete depending on body weight, your chosen sport, how hard and long you train, plus your inherited level of enzyme activity. Some athletes need double this amount of carbohydrate, some need only half. In order to utilize this dietary carbohydrate, muscles must be worked to glycogen depletion so that glycogen synthesis is triggered. Otherwise, excess carbohydrates are converted into fatty acids rather than glycogen. You will need to experiment with how much carbohydrate you can eat without tiring and without losing or gaining weight in the form of body fat. By depleting muscle glycogen during training, muscles subsequently become loaded with more glycogen than they started with. During training this depletion/loading cycle is repeated to maximize muscle glycogen stores prior to an event. It is only the muscles which are exercised that will deplete and load with glycogen, however. The process does not automatically occur in all muscles of the body.

Widespread glycogen-loading is best achieved by doing high repetitions with light weights in the widest selection of exercises possible. Many athletes glycogen-load their leg muscles successfully (e.g. by using a cycle, treadmill, etc.) but are let down by neglecting to exercise their arms, neck, shoulder and even back muscles – these muscles then become depleted of glycogen during the event itself.

It is best to obtain the assistance of a personal trainer to help you glycogen-load successfully.

Carbohydrates Before Exercise

To fuel the event itself you will need to start loading on carbohydrates 3–4 hours before strenuous exercise. This is best achieved in the form of an energy drink containing 100 g of carbohydrate plus obtaining adequate fluid *(see page 316)*.

Carbohydrates During Exercise

Carbohydrates taken during exercise can be a useful source of fuel, but only if your muscle glycogen stores are deficient – because whereas glycogen is in a chemical form that mitochondria can use straight away, glucose taken up from the bloodstream must first be processed by adding a phosphate chemical bond. This is what allows it to drive the regeneration of ATP from ADP.

321

It is much better to load with carbohydrate several hours before the event so the carbohydrate is converted into glycogen which is then already sitting in the muscle cells waiting to be used. Also, if muscle glycogen stores are low before exercise, glucose during exercise is important to prevent muscles turning to protein as an emergency energy source. Even small amounts of glucose have a protein-sparing effect *(see page 311)*.

During a long endurance event you will need 40–90 g carbohydrate (e.g. glucose, maltodextrin) per hour as well as an adequate fluid intake for optimum performance. Research suggests absorption of both is best using 5–10 per cent carbohydrate solutions (sip around a litre per hour depending on level of exercise).

Carbohydrates After Exercise

As soon as you finish exercise, muscle cells must repay any oxygen debt they have incurred. They also start replenishing their diminished stocks of glycogen.

Glycogen synthesis is rapid for the first two hours, slightly less rapid for the next four hours, and occurs at a slow rate for the following 24 hours.

During the first two hours an enzyme (glycogen synthetase) is activated which triggers rapid synthesis of glycogen. This is when you need to hit the carbs in a big way.

It has been found experimentally that an athlete obtaining 225 g glucose polymer in liquid form during the first four hours synthesizes the maximum amount of glycogen. This saturates the enzyme systems, so any more than this does not increase the amount of glycogen synthesized.

So after you have replenished your water intake, start drinking a carbohydrate energy drink which contains high quantities of sugars (10 to 20 g per 100 ml).

You need to maintain a constant, steady intake of carbohydrate (up to 1,000 g in total depending on duration and level of exercise) during the 24 hours after a strenuous event. This is best achieved by eating little and often, for example six small meals spread throughout the day rather than three larger ones, which is the Western norm. This will minimize sugar swings that can trigger insulin fluctuations. If these occur, glycogen synthesis is inhibited and some newly generated glycogen may get broken down.

Complex carbohydrates are best obtained in the form of whole grains (e.g. brown rice, wholewheat pasta, wholemeal bread), legumes (e.g. soybeans, baked beans, lentils, kidney beans), and vegetables (e.g. potatoes, yams).

Your fluid intake must remain high during this glycogen replenishing phase, as each gram of glycogen is associated inside your cells with 2.7 g of water.

After the high intake during the first 24 hours, revert to your normal calorie intake (otherwise you will start putting on fat), but ensure that at least 60 per cent is in the form of carbohydrates.

Dedicated athletes eat as much as 80 per cent of their calories in this form during training periods, which would certainly please the World Health Organization.

FOCUS ON: BODY BUILDERS

Body builders use carbohydrates and glycogen-loading to increase muscle bulk and definition before competition rather than as an energy source.

Starting a week before the event, body builders initially deplete their diet of carbohydrates and increase protein intake to provide around 60–70 per cent of their calories. As soon as glycogen stores are depleted no more can be synthesized due to the lack of dietary carbohydrate. The body preferentially switches to burning fat stores as fuel and the body builder deliberately enters an unpleasant state known as ketosis.

Ketones are a by-product of fat metabolism. They are metabolized with difficulty in the liver and are normally rapidly metabolized in other body tissues. This process requires products of glucose metabolism however, so when carbohydrate intake is low and excess ketones are formed, they spill over into the circulation.

Ketones are an important source of energy in some emergency situations such as during temporary periods of starvation or after prolonged vomiting.

If too many build up in the body, however, they affect the body's acid balance and can cause cell damage. Ketones also affect the brain by acting as false neurotransmitters. This leads to irritability, lethargy and confusion.

Body builders force themselves to work through these feelings by burning up ketones as fuel until they reach the point of exhaustion and maximum glycogen depletion. This is a potentially dangerous situation and should always be done under the strict supervision of a personal trainer and preferably a physician. If ketosis is handled incorrectly, it can be lethal.

Three days before the event, body builders change tactics and increase their carbohydrate intake to 70–80 per cent of energy intake and drop protein right down to only 10 per cent of calories.

Sodium intake is also heavily restricted, with potassium intake raised to compensate. Together with a lowered fluid intake, this encourages mild dehydration to obtain a leaner, more sculpted look.

Ketosis disappears now that carbohydrates are being used as a fuel source, and exercise is kept very light.

Over these three days, muscle glycogen stores rapidly increase from the depleted state so that 2–3 kg in weight are gained.

The combination of glycogen-loading and slight dehydration has to be handled carefully so that water is diverted into the muscles (bound to glycogen) from other body cavities, without causing symptoms of dehydration (dry mouth, dizziness, rapid pulse, increased breathing rate, confusion – even coma).

Some body builders risk their health by taking diuretics or having a sauna to lose even more fluid before the competition. Don't do it!

Body builders are in a highly abnormal physiological state while preparing for competition. Never do this alone without advice from a properly qualified trainer and the input of a sports physician.

DIETARY FATS

The average fat intake in the Western world makes up at least 40 per cent of daily calories. This is far too high. The World Health Organization recommends that fats be reduced to no more than 30 per cent of energy intake – preferably nearer 20 per cent.

For athletes, fat intake should be less than for even the healthiest eating sedentary adult. A certain amount of the right sorts of fats is important, however. The fat (lipid) fraction of our diet supplies us with:

- building blocks for cell membranes
- fatty acids necessary for the central nervous system
- precursors for important hormone-like chemicals called prostaglandins
- substrates for hormone production
- molecules from which to make bile salts
- fat-soluble vitamins A, D, E
- essential fatty acids (linoleic and linolenic acids)
- energy – 9 kcal per g

We lack the enzymes and metabolic pathways needed to convert fat into glucose, therefore dietary fat is shunted into pathways that convert it to body fat – that is, flab.

If carbohydrate is in short supply and fat must be used as an energy source, it must first be mobilized and broken down into fatty acids. This takes time and, in an emergency situation, the body resorts to converting protein stores into glucose to plug the gap.

In addition, the body finds it difficult to mobilize the energy from fat molecules without a plentiful supply of dietary carbohydrate.

Fat in the diet – although ostensibly providing twice as much energy as carbohydrate (9 kcal/g versus 4 kcal/g) is therefore not the best source of energy for anyone – especially athletes. Carbohydrate is the prime energy source.

But athletes do need some fats, and it is important that those

325

they eat should provide the most nutritional benefits.

Fatty acids are made up of chains of carbon and hydrogen atoms. Different fatty acids have chains of different lengths. Fats can be classified into saturated, monounsaturated and polyunsaturated according to their chemical structure. In saturated fats, all the carbon bonds are attached to hydrogen atoms. In mono- and polyunsaturated fats, there are some hydrogen atoms missing. This allows them to interact with the body's metabolism more easily. Monounsaturated fats are only missing one hydrogen atom. Polyunsaturated fats are missing two or more hydrogen atoms.

Most natural fats and oils contain a blend of saturates, monounsaturates and polyunsaturates.

Cholesterol

Cholesterol is an important fat-based structural molecule that is a building block for cell membranes, hormones and bile salts. Two forms of cholesterol exist in the bloodstream:

1. low-density LDL-cholesterol molecules which are small enough to seep into artery walls and trigger hardening and furring up of the arteries (atherosclerosis).
2. high-density HDL-cholesterol molecules that are too large to seep into artery walls and therefore stay in the bloodstream to act as important carrier molecules. They help to mobilize and mop up the risky LDL-cholesterol.

High blood levels of LDL-cholesterol are linked with an increased risk of coronary heart disease, while high levels of HDL-cholesterol are protective (*see* Chapter 11).

It is important to realize that most of the cholesterol in our blood is made in our liver from fats in our diet.

Eating preformed dietary cholesterol (e.g. in egg yolks) has relatively little impact on the amount of cholesterol in our blood.

Saturated Fats

Saturated (hydrogenated) fats tend to be solid at room temperature. They are mainly derived from animal fat and are found in high quantities in cream, butter, egg yolk and red meat.

Saturated fats are converted in the body to harmful LDL-cholesterol. We would be better off without eating any saturated fats, yet they currently make up around 15 per cent of energy intake. Everyone should reduced the intake of saturated fats to less than 10 per cent of calories – preferably zero. This is especially important for optimal sports nutrition.

Unsaturated Fats

Monounsaturated and polyunsaturated fats tend to be liquid at room temperature – i.e. oils. Olive oil is the richest source of monounsaturates, while other vegetable oils such as wheatgerm, sunflowerseed and safflower tend to be rich in polyunsaturates.

Monounsaturated fats help to lower harmful blood LDL-cholesterol levels and raise levels of beneficial high density HDL-cholesterol. Athletes should preferentially use Extra Virgin olive oil or rapeseed oil for cooking and salad dressings.

Polyunsaturated fats are now viewed with some suspicion. They are highly reactive and rapidly oxidize (go rancid) to form carcinogenic (cancer-forming) chemicals. They also affect cell membranes, interfere with cellular transport and possibly promote early ageing.

When polyunsaturates are partially hydrogenated, trans-fatty acids are produced. These are associated with an increased risk of coronary heart disease and may be an even greater health hazard than natural saturated fats.

Trans-fatty acids are also thought to interfere with the way the body handles other essential fatty acids, so that their beneficial effects are not fully realized.

The amount of trans-fatty acids in our diet varies but average consumption is around 5–7 g per day. Some people eat as much

327

as 25–30 g of trans-fatty acids per day, particularly if they use cheap margarine and eat lots of processed foods.

Transfatty acid content of some foods

Food	Total transfatty acids as a % of total fatty acids
Bread	10–28
Cake	10–24
Crackers	3–31
French fries	5–35
Instant puddings	30–36
Hard margarine	18–36
Soft margarine	11–21
Crisps (potato chips)	14–33
Butter	<1

Essential Fats

Two fatty acids cannot be synthesized within the body. These are linoleic and linolenic acid. They must be obtained from dietary sources and are therefore known as essential fatty acids (EFAs).

Both of these essential oils are found in rich quantities in walnuts, pumpkin seeds, soybeans, linseed oil, rapeseed oil and flax oil.

Linoleic acid alone is found in Extra Virgin olive oil and in the oils made from sunflower seeds, almonds, corn, sesame seeds, and safflower.

Linolenic acid alone is found in Evening Primrose oil, starflower oil and borage seed oil, all of which are available as food supplements.

Athletes should follow World Health Organization guidelines and eat at least 30 g of nuts and seeds per day – preferably more.

Fish Oil

Oily fish contain eicosapentanoic acid (EPA) which has been hailed as a miracle substance. It feeds into our metabolic pathways to make certain types of the hormone-like pro-staglandins, which decrease the stickiness of blood. This reduces the risk of blood clots and improves the circulation.

It is now known that EPA is synthesized by minute marine algae called phytoplankton. These are eaten by fish and stored in concentrated form in their body oils. It can also be made in very small quantities in humans. Research suggests that EPA:

- raises beneficial HDL-cholesterol blood levels
- lowers harmful LDL-cholesterol blood levels
- helps prevent death due to coronary thrombosis
- halves the risk of dying from a stroke
- protects against diabetes
- eases the pain and stiffness of arthritis
- helps repair damaged nerves
- improves symptoms of ulcerative colitis
- may have a role in beating cancer by slowing tumour growth and preventing cancer-induced weight loss.

In Denmark, so-called 'healthy bread' containing refined fish oil is on sale. In New Zealand, fish oil is added to milk for health reasons, and in Switzerland many common foods contain added fish oil as a healthy supplement.

The British Nutrition Foundation recommends that the average person increase consumption of oily fish (salmon, herrings, sardines, mackerel, trout) by a factor of 10 – to an equivalent of 300 g (3 portions) mackerel per week. This is even more important for athletes.

Those who do not like fish should seriously consider adding food supplements such as Efamol Marine or Maxepa to their diet.

DIETARY GUIDELINES FOR OPTIMAL SPORTS NUTRITION

- Reduce total fat intake to less than 30 per cent of energy intake – preferably to nearer 20 per cent. Some top athletes follow a diet closer to that of the Japanese, eating only 15 per cent of total calories in the form of fat.

- Eliminate as much saturated fat from your diet as possible.
- Avoid trans-fatty acids.
- Use Extra Virgin olive oil.
- Eat oily fish at least three times per week, or consider taking fish oil supplements.
- Eat at least 30 g of nuts and seeds per day for their essential fatty acid content.
- Consider taking gammalinolenic acid supplements.

NB Gammalinolenic acid (a linoleic acid substitute) and fish oil are available in one prepackaged supplement, *Efamol Marine*.

PROTEIN

Proteins are made up of large chains of building blocks called amino acids. There are 20 amino acids involved in protein formation, of which around half cannot be synthesized in the body in enough quantities to meet day-to-day metabolic needs. These amino acids must come from the diet and are known as the nutritionally essential amino acids:

Amino Acids	Glutamine	**Phenylalanine**
Alanine	Glycine	Proline
Arginine	**Histidine**	Serine
Asparagine	**Isoleucine**	**Threonine**
Aspartic acid	**Leucine**	**Tryptophan**
Cysteine	**Lysine**	**Tyrosine**
Glutamic acid	**Methionine**	**Valine**

Amino acids shown in **bold** are the nutritionally essential ones.

Different proteins contain chains of different amino acids arranged rather like beads on a string. This amino acid order is coded by the DNA within each cell nucleus. In fact, a gene is merely a blueprint dictating the amino acid sequence for the synthesis of a single protein within a cell.

Chains of 2–10 amino acids tend to be called peptides; chains of 10–100 amino acids tend to be called polypeptides, and chains of over 100 amino acids, which are usually folded into complex 3-D shapes, are known as proteins.

There are over 50,000 different proteins and polypeptides in the human body. Some are structural, some act as enzymes to speed metabolic reactions and others form part of the protective immune system.

Over 50 per cent of the dry weight of your body consists of protein. These are constantly being broken down and resynthesized at a turnover rate of around 80–100 g/day. Most muscle protein is renewed every six months – 98 per cent of our total body proteins are renewed within one year.

The average daily need for protein is estimated at around 56 g per day. The average protein intake for men in the UK is higher than this, at 84 g per day.

These figures are misleading where athletes are concerned, for they are more applicable to the average inactive, mainly sedentary man who barely exercises. Athletes who are training hard may need more than twice the dietary protein that sedentary folk need, as their muscles are actively bulking up and also burning protein as emergency fuel.

It is important to realize that a high protein intake does not stimulate muscle growth *per se*. It can only provide building blocks if you are exercising enough to encourage your muscles to bulk.

You need to match your protein intake to your training programme. If you eat more protein than you need to match a light exercise level, it will be converted into carbohydrate plus a waste product containing nitrogen and known as urea. This is excreted from the body via the kidneys. You will be in 'neutral nitrogen balance' because the amount of nitrogen present in your dietary proteins will equal the amount excreted.

If you are exercising enough to stimulate muscle growth, dietary protein will be converted into lean tissue. Your intake of nitrogen (as protein) will be greater than that lost as urea in the urine, as some has been converted into muscle mass. Your nitrogen balance is then said to be positive.

331

If you exercise but eat too little protein, your muscle bulk may reduce rather than increase in size. Muscle proteins, like other body proteins, are constantly being turned over and will be broken down as normal. By eating too little protein, however, the amino acids needed to resynthesize protein are in short supply. Your nitrogen balance is negative as you are losing more nitrogen from your body (in the form of urea derived from muscles) than you have obtained from protein in your diet. This will impair your performance potential.

Athletes training for two hours per day need around 1.1–1.4 g protein per kg body weight per day just to maintain nitrogen balance, depending on the intensity of exercise.

Those doing three hours of training per day may need 1.2–1.5 g/kg/day depending on how hard they are pushing themselves.

Those doing five hours of intense exercise per day may need up to 1.8 g/kg/day just to maintain nitrogen balance.

Body builders in training may obtain as much as 2–3.5 g protein per kg of body weight per day. They are training hard to bulk up their muscles, and need protein to provide the necessary building blocks. Unfortunately, they also cut back on carbohydrates to alter their muscle glycogen content *(see page 323)*.

But can increasing your protein intake actually increase your potential to put on muscle bulk? Only if you are exercising your muscles hard enough to encourage bulking.

There is evidence that athletes training intensively for over three hours per day will put on extra muscle bulk if they have a higher (i.e. adequate) protein intake. In one experiment, healthy males were divided into two groups and fed either 1.4 g protein/kg/day or 2.8 g protein/kg/day, with total calorie intakes for both groups equalling 3,600 kcal.

A 40-day intensive exercise regime followed; by its end, those on the lower protein intake had gained an average of 1.21 kg lean body mass. Those in the higher protein intake had gained as much as 3.28 kg lean mass.

This should not be interpreted to mean that eating more protein will automatically increase muscle bulk. What it implies is that the lower protein intake was inadequate to match the intensive exercise regime, but in order to allow muscle bulk to reach its full potential, the higher protein intake was needed.

It is important not to eat too much protein. Excess dietary protein (above your body's needs) is converted into carbohydrate and, ultimately, if you are eating more calories than you need, it may even end up as flab.

Excess protein intake also generates excess blood urea, which can make you feel lethargic and generally unwell.

Try to obtain dietary protein from eating fish, white meat, wholegrains, nuts, seeds and beans rather than eating a lot of red meat and dairy products which (apart from egg white) are also high in saturated fat.

Athletes on an intensive exercise training regime will also need protein supplements. These are available as intact proteins, partially digested (hydrolysed) peptides, and as free amino acids.

There is evidence to suggest that the hydrolysates (dipeptides and tripeptides) may have additional (anabolic) actions in the body to promote muscle bulking.

19

VITAMINS AND MEN'S HEALTH

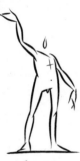 Vitamins are essential organic substances that have specific metabolic functions in the human body. Most cannot be synthesized in sufficient quantities to fulfil biochemical needs and therefore must be obtained from dietary sources.

In many cases vitamins are required in very small amounts; too much is as harmful as not enough. Athletes have a higher vitamin need than sedentary males, as their basal metabolic rate is higher.

A varied wholefood diet is critical to provide as many vitamins as possible from dietary sources, but in many cases supplements are needed too.

The following overview of vitamins (minerals are discussed in the next chapter) gives the recommended daily amounts required for health in both sedentary and intensively training males. Dietary sources are listed for each nutrient reviewed.

To give you an idea of how much of each vitamin the average diet provides, the table below shows the average intake of each vitamin for British men aged between 16 and 64 years. Average intakes are shown for males who take food supplements as well.

Against these, the UK/EC Recommended Daily Amount of each nutrient (RDA) is given.

Average UK dietary intake

Nutrient	Males (mean)	Males taking supplements	EC/UK RDAs
Vitamin A	1186 mcg	2244 mcg	800 mcg
Betacarotene	2.4 mg	2.8 mg	(*)
Thiamin (B$_1$)	1.7 mg	5.5 mg	1.4 mg
Riboflavin (B$_2$)	2.1 mg	4.8 mg	1.6 mg
Niacin (B$_3$)	39.5 mg	55 mg	18 mg
Pantothenic acid	6.2 mg	10.2 mg	6 mg
Vitamin B$_6$	2.5 mg	5 mg	2 mg
Vitamin B$_{12}$	7.1 mcg	9.3 mcg	1 mcg
Folate	308 mcg	355 mcg	200 mcg
Biotin	38.5 mcg	45.3 mcg	0.15 mg
Vitamin C	64.8 mg	179.6 mg	60 mg
Vitamin D	3.4 mcg	8.1 mg	5 mcg
Vitamin E	9.7 mg	32.4 mg	10 mg

*No EC RDA, but National Cancer Institute suggest a minimum intake of 6 mg of betacarotene per day. Sources: The Dietary and Nutritional Survey of British Adults (OPCS) 1990. HMSO Publication SS1241.

At first glance it would appear that most men not taking supplements are obtaining RDAs of most vitamins except betacarotene and possibly the important antioxidant vitamin E.

But RDAs are not recommended amounts for each individual – we all vary greatly in our needs, according to our metabolic rate, our diet and the amount of exercise we take. Athletes usually need higher vitamin intakes than these.

RDAs are designed solely to compare populations and ensure that, in general, people are getting enough of the nutrients we all need. Athletes will need more of many of these vitamins, merely because they are making more demands on their metabolism – the reactions for which vitamins are essential.

The other important point is that an average is only an average: half of the population will be getting more than the average intakes found in the government survey quoted above, and half will be getting less. For example, although the average vitamin C intake is 64.8 mg per day, the observed intake range is wide, with some men only obtaining 20 mg/day while others get as much as 170 mg/day from their diet.

It is estimated that 60 per cent of the British adult population are not getting the recommended amounts of vitamin C (60 mg/day) from their diet.

VITAMIN A

Preformed vitamin A is only found in animal products. It is fat soluble, stored in the liver and most of us have enough stores to last at least one year.

Vitamin A is essential for vision, healthy moist eyes, sexual reproduction, the integrity of cell membranes and for normal growth and development.

- EC/UK RDA for adult males: 800 mcg (micrograms) of Vitamin A per day.
- US Recommended Daily Allowance (RDA): 1,000 mcg per day.
  - There is no evidence that athletes need more than this amount.
  - Most men in the Western world already have a vitamin A intake greater than this.
- Average dietary intake for British males: 1,186 mcg/day. Observed intakes range from 190–6,560 mcg from food sources.
- Foods rich in vitamin A include:
  - kidneys
  - eggs
  - milk
  - cheese
  - yoghurt
  - butter
  - oily fish.
- Margarine sold in the UK is also fortified with vitamin A by law.
- On average, men obtain 14 per cent of dietary preformed vitamin A from milk and milk products, 14 per cent from fat spreads, 6 per cent from cereal products, 4 per cent from eggs and egg products and a massive 55 per cent from liver products.
- Too much vitamin A is poisonous, causing symptoms of nausea, headache, visual disturbances, skin sloughing, coma and even death. It is important not to take supplements containing high doses of vitamin A. It is much safer to obtain your requirements in the form of the pro-vitamin, betacarotene.

Betacarotene

Various vitamin A-like compounds (carotenoids) are found in vegetables. Unlike vitamin A, these are water soluble and cannot build up in the body to cause harm, as whatever the body does not need is flushed out through the kidneys.

The most important carotenoid, betacarotene, consists of two molecules of vitamin A joined together. When body stores of vitamin A are low, some molecules of betacarotene are split to yield vitamin A. Zinc is essential for this reaction, so if zinc levels are low, there may be an associated deficiency of vitamin A.

When vitamin A stores are high, betacarotene stays as it is – and has its own important functions in protecting against disease. It is a powerful antioxidant, helping to overcome the damage to cells caused by free radicals (*see* Chapter 21) and protects the male sperm.

- EC/UK RDA: none.
- US recommended intake (as suggested by the US National Cancer Institute): a minimum of 6 mg per day to reduce the risk of cancer.
- Research in the US on 22,000 male doctors has also shown that men with the highest intake of betacarotene reduced their risk of coronary heart disease by as much as 25 per cent.
- UK average dietary intake: 2.4 mg/day. This is way below NCI recommendations, although observed intakes range from 0.2–7.5 mg from food sources.
- Foods rich in betacarotene include:
  - dark green leafy vegetables (e.g. spinach, broccoli)
  - yellow-orange fruit (e.g. carrots, apricots, mangoes, red and yellow peppers and sweet potatoes).
- On average, men obtain 69 per cent of dietary betacarotene from vegetables and 13 per cent from meat and meat products, with the remaining amounts coming from cereal products, fruits, nuts and fat spreads.

VITAMIN B$_1$ (THIAMIN)

Thiamin is needed for the production of energy from carbohydrate and for the synthesis of some amino acids. It also plays a role in healthy nerve conduction. Athletes in training therefore need more of this vitamin than the average sedentary male to convert blood sugar into biological energy, and for the maintenance of healthy muscles.

Thiamin is water soluble and is not stored to any great extent in the body. An adequate daily supply is essential to burn the increased amounts of carbohydrate that athletes eat. Drinking large amounts of coffee or tea destroys this vitamin.

- EC/UK RDA: 1.4 mg/day
- US RDA: 1.5 mg/day
- UK average dietary intake: 1.7 mg/day. Observed intakes range from 0.8–2.9 mg from food sources.

   Some sports experts advise athletes in training (on a high carbohydrate diet) to get as much as 50–200 mg thiamin per day to maintain acceptable levels of this vitamin. There is no evidence that excess thiamin is toxic.
- Foods rich in vitamin B$_1$ include:
  wheat germ
  wholegrain products
  oatmeal
  yeast extract
  brown rice
  meats
  seafood
  pulses
  nuts.
- Highly milled grains (e.g. polished white rice) and those that have been in storage for any length of time will lose their thiamin content.
- On average, men get 38 per cent of dietary thiamin from cereal products, 26 per cent from vegetables (mainly potatoes), 19 per cent from meats and 8 per cent from milk products.

VITAMIN B₂ (RIBOFLAVIN)

Riboflavin is another water-soluble vitamin essential for smooth metabolic functioning. It is known as 'the exerciser's friend' as it is involved in the production of the energy within mitochondria *(see page 310)*.

It is also involved in the metabolism of carbohydrate, fatty acids and protein. As such, an adequate supply is essential for athletes, who require more than sedentary men. If riboflavin is in short supply, oxygen consumption goes down, thereby impairing performance.

- EC/UK RDA: 1.6 mg/day.
- US RDA: 1.7 mg/day.
  Those who exercise moderately probably need a total of at least 2–2.5 mg riboflavin per day. Some sports nutritionists recommend intakes of 25 mg to 200 mg for athletes in full training, in order to maintain personal performance. There is no evidence that excess riboflavin will boost performance, or that it is toxic.
- UK average dietary intake: 2.1 mg/day. Observed intakes vary from 1–3.6 mg from food sources.
- Foods rich in riboflavin include:
  liver
  milk
  cheese
  yoghurt
  yeast extract
  eggs
  wheat bran
  green leafy vegetables
  mushrooms
  fruits
  bread
  cereals
  meats.
- On average, men get 26 per cent of dietary riboflavin from milk and milk products (especially cheese), 22 per cent from meat and meat products and 21 per cent from cereals. 8 per cent of intake comes from beer.

VITAMIN B₃ (NIACIN; NIACINAMIDE; NICOTINAMIDE; NICOTINIC ACID)

Niacin is another water-soluble vitamin that plays an important role in the formation of metabolic enzymes and energy production. It is essential for producing energy from glycogen, for the oxidation of fatty acids and for tissue respiration. As such, athletes require more niacin than sedentary men.

It comes in several forms and can also be synthesized in the body from the essential amino acid, tryptophan.

- EC/UK RDA: 18 mg/day.
- US National Research Council recommended intake: 19 mg/day.

  Some sports nutritionists recommend that athletes in training need as much as 30–100 mg per day (mostly in the form of nicotinamide) to maintain adequate levels. Don't take more than this unless under medical supervision, and stick to nicotinamide which does not cause flushing. Intakes of over 30 mg niacin and intakes above 100 mg nicotinic acid dilate blood vessels, leading to skin redness, burning, tingling and itching – the so-called 'niacin flush'. This is not dangerous in itself, but a few people also suffer nausea, headache, muscle cramps and diarrhoea. Lowered blood pressure and pulse may also induce feelings of faintness.

  Doses above 500 mg niacin equivalents per day are toxic and can lead to liver damage.
- UK average dietary intake: 40 mg/day. Observed intakes vary from 21–62 mg from food sources.
- Foods rich in vitamin B₃ include:
  lean meat
  fish
  poultry
  yeast extract
  peanuts
  bran
  beans
  milk
  whole grains.

- On average, men get 34 per cent of dietary niacin from meat and meat products, 27 per cent from cereals, 10 per cent from vegetables and 9 per cent from milk and milk products.

Theories that megadoses of niacin will boost athletic performance are untrue. There was an initial flurry of excitement at findings that high intakes of niacin (3–10 g daily!) helped to mobilize and burn glycogen more quickly as a fuel.

Unfortunately, this effect also blocks the use of fatty acids as a fuel, leading to rapid glycogen depletion. Performance is therefore actually impaired.

Sixty mg of the amino acid tryptophan is equivalent to 1 mg of preformed dietary niacin. Niacin equivalents are estimated by adding preformed niacin intake plus one sixtieth of tryptophan intake.

Interestingly, it is estimated that intakes of tryptophan among sedentary Western adults is more than adequate to meet niacin needs even if no preformed niacin were available in the diet.

VITAMIN B5 (PANTOTHENIC ACID)

Pantothenic acid is also a water-soluble vitamin essential for many energy-yielding metabolic reactions involving carbohydrates, fats and protein. It is an important component of Co-enzyme Q (an enzyme-helping factor responsible for many metabolic reactions), and is also required for the synthesis of glucose and fatty acids within the body.

- EC/UK RDA: 6 mg/day.
- US RDA: 6 mg/day.
- UK average dietary intake for men: 6.2 mg/day. Observed intakes range from 3–10 mg from food sources.

  Active athletes use up to four times the daily energy of sedentary men and therefore require a higher intake of pantothenic acid. Some sports nutritionists suggest that athletes in training obtain 20–200 mg pantothenic acid per day to reduce the build-up of lactic acid and maximize oxygen consumption. There is no evidence that excess is toxic.

Claims that pantothenic acid can boost athletic performance are interesting. In one study, highly conditioned long-distance runners were given 1 g of pantothenic acid daily for 14 days. Another group was given an inactive placebo and their performance (using a treadmill) was compared to that of the first group. No differences were noted.

In another trial, however, long-distance runners were given 2 g pantothenic acid daily for two weeks and another group received a placebo. Differences were found here. Those receiving megadoses of pantothenic acid experienced a 17 per cent reduction in lactic acid build-up and consumed 8 per cent less oxygen to perform an equivalent amount of work.

In view of the conflicting evidence, more research is awaited before definite claims are made.

Pantothenic acid derives its name from the Greek meaning found 'on all quarters'. It is widely distributed in nature and found in almost every food source, especially meat, eggs and whole-grain cereals. Perhaps the richest source is royal jelly.

VITAMIN B₆ (PYRIDOXINE)

Vitamin B_6 is needed for the proper functioning of over 60 enzymes and is involved in the synthesis and metabolism of nucleic acids, amino acids and proteins.

It is also involved in the burning of glycogen as fuel.

- EC/UK RDA: 2 mg/day
- US RDA: 2 mg/day
- UK average dietary intake: 2.5 mg/day. Observed intakes vary from 1–4.5 mg.

  Some sports nutritionists recommend that athletes ensure an intake of 10 mg to 50 mg per day. More than this is not recommended. Supplements providing 100 mg to 500 mg vitamin B_6 per tablet are potentially dangerous if used without medical

supervision.
- Foods rich in vitamin B_6 include:
  meat
  whole-grain cereals
  nuts
  yeast extract
  vegetables.

Excessive vitamin B_6 (several hundreds of mg/day) taken over several weeks or months can produce symptoms of nerve damage (tingling, burning, shooting pains, pins and needles, clumsiness, numbness, even partial paralysis), depression, headache, tiredness, bloatedness and irritability. These symptoms are only partially helped by eliminating B_6 supplements from the diet.

More modest doses (100 mg/day for several months) cause less serious nerve damage, resulting in tingling sensations in the fingers and toes that goes away once supplements are discontinued.

VITAMIN B_{12} (COBALAMIN)

Vitamin B_{12} is an essential component of several coenzymes. It cooperates with another vitamin, folate, during the synthesis of genetic material (DNA) – a process that occurs continuously during muscular development and red blood cell formation. Deficiency of either vitamin leads to the formation of abnormal cells that are larger than they should be (megablastosis). Vitamin B_{12} also plays a role in the formation of healthy nerve sheaths (myelin).

- EC/UK RDA: 1 mcg/day. Some countries recommend an adult intake of 3 mcg/day.
- UK average dietary intake: 7 mcg/day. Observed variations range from 2–23 mcg/day.
  There is little evidence that athletes need much more than this observed average intake – although some nutritionists

343

recommend intakes of up to 50 mcg for everyone, athlete or not. Most adults who eat meat products obtain at least 5 micrograms vitamin B_{12} per day.

- Some athletes receive megashots of vitamin B_{12} injections before competitions. There is no evidence that this practice is efficacious, although it does seem to be safe.
- Foods rich in vitamin B_{12} include:
  liver
  fish (especially sardines)
  meat
  eggs
  milk
  cheese.
- No vegetables are known consistently to contain vitamin B_{12} – an important point for vegetarian, especially vegan (lacto-vegetarian) men. Preparations of vitamin B_{12} made by bacterial fermentation – and therefore acceptable to vegetarians – are readily available.

Vitamin B_{12} deficiency is fairly common, but this is usually due to malabsorption from the intestine rather than dietary lack. It can result in pernicious anaemia. This is triggered when the body stops making *intrinsic factor* – a substance secreted in the stomach which is needed for the absorption of vitamin B_{12} lower down the intestinal tract.

FOLATE (FOLIC ACID)

Folate is involved in the formation of coenzymes that control amino acid and sugar metabolism. It is needed for the synthesis of nucleic acids during cell division, and is vital for red blood cell formation.

Body folate stores are small and deficiency develops quickly – it is probably the most widespread vitamin deficiency in industrialized countries.

- EC/UK RDA: 200 mcg/day.

- US RDA: 200 mcg/day (300 mcg/day until recently)
- UK average daily intake for men: 308 mcg/day. Observed intakes vary from 145–555 mcg.
- There is no evidence that moderate supplementation with folic acid is harmful. There are two potential problems, however:

  1. taking folate supplements alone may mask a vitamin B_{12} deficiency, and the imbalance can lead to spinal cord damage.
  2. anticonvulsant drugs to control epilepsy work by increasing folate metabolism (which can trigger deficiency). Taking folate supplements (greater than 1 g/day) may antagonize the beneficial effects of anticonvulsant drugs and increase the frequency of epileptic fits. Epileptic men on medication should discuss supplementation with their neurologist.

- Some sports nutritionists suggest that active athletes need 800–4,800 mcg folate to maintain adequate body supplies and optimum performance. This is only safe as long as pernicious anaemia due to vitamin B_{12} deficiency or malabsorption has been ruled out.
- Foods rich in vitamin B include:
  fish (especially sardines and oysters)
  meats (especially liver, kidney and rabbit)
  dairy products
  wholegrain cereals
  oranges
  nuts
  yeast.
- On average, men get most dietary folate from dark green vegetables (35 per cent), bread and flour products (26 per cent), meat products (10 per cent), milk products (9 per cent) and fruit (6 per cent).

NB Prolonged boiling destroys much of the folate present in green leafy vegetables.

345

BIOTIN

Biotin is a water-soluble vitamin. It acts as a co-factor for several enzymes involved in the synthesis of fatty acids, purine nucleotides (building blocks for DNA) and in the metabolism of some amino acids (valine, isoleucine and leucine). It is also essential for the formation of new glucose within the body and, as such, is especially important for athletes.

Biotin is widely distributed in food and is also synthesized by bacteria in our own intestines. The amount excreted in faeces is up to six times higher than that ingested in the diet. Deficiency is therefore rare except in people who eat large amounts of raw egg white – an important point for body-builders to note. Egg white contains a protein called *avidin* which binds to biotin synthesized in the digestive tract and prevents its absorption. Avidin is denatured by cooking, however, and loses its ability to bind biotin.

Men eating a poor diet who are also on long-term antibiotic treatment may be at risk of biotin deficiency, as may those following very low-calorie weight loss diets. Biotin deficiency leads to flaking skin, wasted muscles and hair loss.

- EC/UK RDA: 150 mcg/day (intakes between 10 and 200 mcg are thought to be both safe and adequate).
- US RDA: 100 mcg/day (until recently it was 300 mcg).
- UK average daily intake: 38.5 mcg/day. Intakes range from 15–70 mcg/day.
  Although apparently low, these intakes do not seem to cause deficiency, presumably because of the dietary top up of biotin manufactured by intestinal tract bacteria.
- Some sports nutritionist suggest athletes in intensive training require 300–5,000 mcg/day to optimize protein and glucose synthesis. There is no evidence that excess biotin either improves athletic performance, or that it is toxic.
- Foods rich in biotin include:
  liver
  sardines
  egg yolk

whole grains (especially soy)
nuts
milk
vegetables.

VITAMIN C

Vitamin C is a water-soluble vitamin essential for the synthesis of collagen – a major structural protein important for combating sports injury – and for the synthesis of adrenaline and noradrenaline. These are important neurotransmitters with several roles in the body, including the fight-or-flight reaction.

Vitamin C also acts as an antioxidant to mop up dangerous free radicals produced by metabolic reactions. As such, an active sportsperson with a raised metabolic rate is likely to need more vitamin C than a sedentary male. Vitamin C is an important component of semen.

Vitamin C has an additional important role – that of regenerating the lipid-soluble antioxidant vitamin E from its oxidized form back into its protective, reduced form *(see page 369)*.

- Current recommendations for vitamin C intake vary widely:
  - The Netherlands: 80 mg/day
  - US RDA: 60 mg/day.
  - EC/UK RDA: 60 mg/day.
- Smokers need at least 100 mg vitamin C per day to mop up the excess free radicals generated by their habit.
- Some sports nutritionists suggest athletes need as much as 2–12 g per day. There is little evidence of toxicity as, being water soluble, any excess vitamin C is voided in the urine. This seems to protect against bladder cancer. Certainly people who take megadoses of vitamin C seem to live longer and have a significantly reduced risk of coronary heart disease and cancer. A few people notice symptoms of diarrhoea if they take too much vitamin C.
- UK average dietary UK intake: 64.8 mg/day. Observed average intakes vary widely: 19–171 mg/day. It can be estimated that

347

60 per cent of adults do not obtain the EC recommended amount of 60 mg/day.
- Foods rich in vitamin C include:
blackcurrants
guavas
citrus fruits
mangoes
kiwi fruit
green peppers
strawberries
green sprouting vegetables (e.g. broccoli, sprouts, watercress) and potatoes.
- On average, we obtain 50 per cent of our daily intake from vegetables (19 per cent from potatoes), 17 per cent from fruit juice drinks and 14 per cent from fruits and nuts.

Large doses of vitamin C assist the absorption of dietary iron but may have adverse effects on the copper status of men. Whether or not this is significant is unknown. It is also possible that taking vitamin C with inorganic selenium *(see page 363)* might make it less easily absorbed. Use selenium derived from yeast instead.

Vitamin C and the Common Cold

Vitamin C is one of the most popular winter supplements, as many men appreciate its benefits in relieving symptoms of the common cold. Studies show that taking vitamin C at a dose of 1 to 6 g daily can significantly reduce the duration of a cold by over 20 per cent. Interestingly, for certain groups of males – especially school children and students, and men doing heavy physical exercise – vitamin C can also reduce the risk of catching a cold in the first place by almost a third. Studies involving military troops under training and participants in a 90-km running race found that taking 600 mg to 1 g vitamin C per day halved the risk of developing cold symptoms even when exposed to a cold virus.

Researchers are not certain how vitamin C works, but believe its powerful antioxidant action mops up the inflammatory chemicals produced during a viral infection, which improves symptoms and hastens healing. If you find high-dose vitamin C too acidic, take Ester-C instead. Ester-C contains the active breakdown products produced in the body when standard vitamin C is metabolized, and is non-acidic. It is sometimes described as 'body-ready' and has the additional benefits of entering the bloodstream more quickly than normal vitamin C and also stays in the body for longer. Ester-C is included in several mainstream brands of multinutrient supplement – just check the labels to find it.

VITAMIN D

Vitamin D stimulates synthesis of a calcium transport protein in the lining of the small intestines and is essential for the absorption of dietary calcium. Adequate amounts of vitamin D are needed for calcium balance and to maintain healthy bones and teeth.

Most of our vitamin D is synthesized from a cholesterol-like molecule in the skin due to the action of short wavelength ultraviolet light. Blood levels of vitamin D are naturally highest at the end of summer and lowest at the end of winter. People living in high altitudes, who cover up their skin in sunlight or who stay indoors all the time may have insufficient exposure to UV light to synthesize required amounts. Dietary sources are then critical.

- EC/UK RDA: 5 mcg/day.
- UK average dietary intake: 3.4 mcg/day. Intakes vary from 0.5–10 mcg.
- There is no evidence that athletes need more than 10 mcg per day. Amounts only five times this can be toxic. Those taking more than 250 mcg of vitamin D supplements develop high blood calcium levels leading to symptoms of thirst, anorexia, excess urine production and kidney stones. Toxicity only occurs

through too much oral intake, not through exposure to sun, where synthesis is self-limiting.
- Foods rich in vitamin D include:
oily fish (sardines, herring, mackerel, salmon)
tuna
fortified margarine
eggs
whole milk
butter.
- On average, men obtain 32 per cent of dietary vitamin D from fortified fat spreads, 22 per cent from oily fish and 22 per cent from cereal products.

NB 1 mcg vitamin D (cholecalciferol) = 40 iu

VITAMIN E

Vitamin E functions mainly as an antioxidant, mopping up dangerous free radicals formed during metabolism (*see* Chapter 21) that damage cells. Vitamin E is important in protecting body fat stores, blood cholesterol, lipid cell membranes and dietary fats from damaging oxidation. The more fats in your diet – especially healthy ones derived from olive oil and oily fish, the more vitamin E you need.

Vitamin E also has a strengthening effect on muscle fibres and is an important component of semen *(see page 71).*

- EC/UK RDA: 10 mg/day
- US RDA: 10 mg/day
- It is estimated that 98 per cent of adults obtain less than this.
- UK average dietary intake: 9.7 mg/day. Observed intakes vary from 3.5–19.5 mg.
- Many experts now believe a daily intake of at least 40 mg to 50 mg vitamin E is needed to provide adequate protection against free radical damage causing coronary heart disease and cancer. This means taking supplements – though they must be of natural source vitamin E (d-alpha-tocopherol), not synthetic

dl-alphatocopherol which is less biologically potent.

- Some sports nutritionists recommend that athletes obtain as much as 400–2,000 mg vitamin E per day. Vitamin C is required to regenerate vitamin E once it has performed its antioxidant role, therefore adequate supplies of both vitamins are essential. Studies suggest that athletes who supplement with vitamin C and vitamin E show a 25 per cent reduction in soft tissue damage, with muscle and red blood cell membranes sustaining less oxidative damage from free radicals generated during exercise. Muscles also seem to recover and regenerate more quickly following exercise.
- Foods rich in vitamin E include:
  vegetable oils – of which wheatgerm oil is the richest
  avocados
  margarine
  eggs
  butter
  wholemeal cereals
  seeds
  nuts
  seafood
  broccoli.

Vitamin E content of various oils

Oil	Level of vitamin E (mg/100 g)
Wheatgerm	136
Sunflower	49
Safflower	40
Palm	33
Rape seed	22
Codliver	20
Corn	17
Peanut	15
Olive	5

20

MINERALS, TRACE ELEMENTS AND MEN'S HEALTH

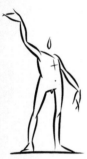

Carbohydrate, fats, proteins and vitamins are all based on the element carbon, and are known as *organic* substances. Minerals do not contain carbon and are said to be *inorganic*.

Inorganic substances of which we need more than 100 mg in our diet are referred to as minerals. Those needed in amounts much less than 100 mg are referred to as trace elements.

Minerals and trace elements are just as important as organic nutrients to both sedentary and active men.

The table below shows the average amount of each mineral nutrient British men (aged 16 and 64) obtain from their diet. Against this is shown the UK/EC recommended daily amount (RDA) for each mineral. The average male's iron intake is lower than the new EC/UK RDA.

The dietary intakes quoted in the table are only averages (mean). Some men will be getting more, others less. In general, mineral and trace element deficiencies are more likely to occur than vitamin deficiencies, especially in parts of the world where soil mineral levels are poor. Mineral supplements are sometimes appropriate, for even if only one mineral is in short supply, the metabolism of other nutrients is affected.

Average UK dietary intake

	Males (mean)	EC/UK RDA
Minerals		
Calcium	937 mg	800 mg
Chloride	5179 mg	2500 mg
Magnesium	323 mg	300 mg
Phosphorus	1452 mg	800 mg
Potassium	3187 mg	3500 mg
Sodium	3376 mg	1600 mg
Trace Elements		
Chromium	25 mcg*	
Copper	1.59 mg	1.2 mg
Iodine	237 mcg	150 mcg
Iron	13.9 mg	14 mg
Manganese	1.4 mg*	
Molybdenum	50–400 mcg*	
Selenium		
Zinc	11.4 mg	15 mg

*No RDAs, but these intakes are deemed both safe and adequate.
Source: The Dietary and Nutritional Survey of British Adults (OPCS) HMSO Publication SS1241.

CALCIUM

Calcium is needed for the growth and development of strong, healthy bones and teeth. Ninety-nine per cent of the body's stores are in the bones, with the other 1 per cent playing a crucial role in blood clotting, muscle contraction, nerve conduction, the production of energy, and immunity.

A dietary deficiency at any stage in life results in raids being made on bone stores which significantly increases the risk of developing osteoporosis (brittle bones) in later life.

In general, exercise strengthens bones, and due to increased mineralization the calcium needs of athletes increase. If the diet is relatively poor in calcium, sports training may result in inadequately mineralized bones, weakened bones and stress fractures.

- EC/UK RDA: 800 mg/day.
- US RDA: 1,200 mg/day.
  The National Osteoporosis Society is lobbying for these recommendations to be raised to at least 1000 mg per day for adult men.
- UK average dietary intake: 400–1,600 mg/day.
- Some sports nutritionists suggest that athletes need supplements of 400–1,600 mg/day. Intakes of up to 2,500 mg/day seem safe, although higher intakes may result in kidney stones.
- Foods rich in calcium include:
  milk
  yoghurt
  cheese
  green vegetables
  oranges
  bread.

Vitamin D is needed for absorption of calcium from the digestive tract. Usually only a small fraction of dietary calcium is taken up (typically less than 40 per cent); the remainder is lost in bowel motions.

It is relatively easy to increase calcium intake. Drinking an extra pint of skimmed or semi-skimmed milk per day provides as much calcium as whole milk (700 mg) but without the additional saturated fat.

By law in the UK, white and brown flour must be fortified with calcium – but this does not apply to wholemeal flour.

Men with a tendency to kidney stones should avoid calcium supplements unless medically supervised.

NB High levels of calcium in the digestive tract interfere with iron uptake.

CHLORIDE

Chloride is a negatively charged electrolyte that, together with sodium (outside the cells) and potassium (inside the cells), controls our fluid and electrolyte balance.

Most adults in the Western World obtain too much salt (sodium chloride). This is a mineral on which you need to cut down, rather than worry about deficiency.

Don't add table salt to food, avoid salted snacks and try not to add salt during cooking either.

MAGNESIUM

Magnesium is the third commonest mineral inside body cells after potassium and phosphorus. It is an integral part of over 300 enzymes and is needed for every major biological process, from the synthesis of protein and nucleic acids to glucose metabolism, muscle contraction and energy production. It is essential for burning carbohydrate as a fuel.

- EC/UK RDA: 300 mg/day.
- US National Research Council recommendation: 350 mg/day.
- UK average daily intake: 323 mg/day. Intakes range from 150–550 mg.
- Active sportspeople need more magnesium than sedentary men to assist muscle contraction and to replace magnesium lost in sweat. Deficiency can cause poor appetite, tiredness, muscle cramps, tics, twitching and weakness.
- Some sports nutritionists prescribe magnesium supplements of 400–1,000 mg per day for athletes in full training. There is no evidence of toxicity at doses of up to 6,000 mg per day, so long as kidneys and heart are functioning normally.
- Foods rich in magnesium include:
  dark green, leafy vegetables
  nuts
  seafood
  seaweed
  soya beans
  meat
  eggs
  dairy products
  wholegrains.

- Drinking water from hard-water areas is another important source.

A diet high in refined and processed foods will be deficient in magnesium as well as other important minerals, vitamins and fibre.

PHOSPHORUS

Ninety per cent of body phosphorus is associated with calcium in the bones. The remainder forms essential, energy-rich molecules (e.g. ATP, ADP) that are instrumental in controlling metabolic reactions concerned with burning fuel.

- EC/UK RDA: 800 mg/day.
- Most adult men obtain more than this. The only men who may develop deficiency are those using antacids containing aluminium hydroxide. This impairs absorption of phosphates from the digestive tract.

Sodium phosphate supplements do seem to improve athletic performance. Tests with endurance athletes (e.g. cyclists) showed that megadose supplements of sodium phosphate (4 g per day) for three days prior to an event decreased lactic acid accumulation, increased oxygen consumption by 11 per cent and lengthened by 20 per cent the amount of time before they felt exhausted. Other studies suggest that sodium phosphate supplements can increase maximal power output by up to 17 per cent.

Potassium phosphate is currently being researched to see if it has the same effect. Calcium phosphate has no beneficial ergogenic effect at all. Phosphate fuel products which boost athletes' intake are now available.

POTASSIUM

Potassium is the main positively charged electrolyte found inside cells. It balances the sodium ions found in the extracellular fluid and is essential for muscle contraction, nerve conduction and for the production of nucleic acids, proteins and energy. Deficiency causes fatigue, weakness and muscle pains, although this usually only occurs when taking non-potassium-sparing diuretic drugs. Potassium chloride is considered a healthier alternative to sodium chloride. Diets high in potassium and low in sodium are linked with a lower risk of high blood pressure and stroke.

- EC/UK RDA: 3,500 mg/day.
- UK average dietary intake: 3,187 mg/day. Observed intakes range from 1,700–4,800 mg.

Athletes need more potassium than sedentary men. They can lose up to 800 mg potassium in sweat per day, and studies show that many athletes are potassium deficient.

Intakes are easily maintained by eating seafood and plenty of fresh fruit and vegetables. Avoid processed, canned or any prepacked foods as these usually have a reversed sodium: potassium ratio. Stick to fresh wholefoods instead.

Sports nutritionists prescribe potassium supplements of 100–500 mg per day for some athletes – although a medium-sized banana would provide the same amount.

SODIUM

Sodium is the main positively charged electrolyte outside of cells. A pump in the cell membrane maintains high potassium levels inside cells to offset the sodium in the extracellular fluid.

- EC/UK RDA: 1,600 mg/day.
- UK average intake: 3,380 mg/day. Intakes range from 1,550–5,600 mg.

Some Western men eat as much as 12 g salt (sodium chloride) per day, which is putting health at risk through rising blood pressure and increased chance of a stroke *(see page 203)*.

357

Most athletes do not need sodium supplements, even in the form of electrolyte drinks. Sweating makes you lose more water than sodium, and after a good work out you will have a higher relative proportion of sodium to water than before you started. You need water first *(see page 317)* and then carbohydrates *(see page 322)* but not salt.

Athletes should never take salt tablets – just the reverse. Don't add salt to food during the cooking or at the table. This will knock around 3 g off your daily salt intake. Concentrate on potassium instead. Apart from anything else, your lifetime's exposure to salt is linked with your risk of developing high blood pressure.

CHROMIUM

Chromium is essential for the normal metabolism of glucose, insulin and fatty acids, and for muscle growth. Adequate intakes are therefore vital for athletes.

Chromium is needed in trace amounts to form an organic complex called Glucose Tolerance Factor (GTF). This contains vitamin B_3 (niacin) and three amino acids as well as chromium. It is essential for the interaction between the hormone insulin and its cell wall receptors.

- US National Research Council suggested intake: 50–200 mcg/day.
- The optimum chromium intake is unknown.
- The average intake is below 50 mcg and it is thought that only 2 per cent is in an absorbable form. Deficiency is therefore common and seems to be associated with poor glucose tolerance, as is seen in diabetes.

Body stores of chromium are rapidly depleted by following a high carbohydrate/sugar diet and through exercise. Running significantly increases the urinary loss of chromium. Athletes therefore need more than sedentary men.

Chromium in the form of picolinate has been shown to help

muscle cells take up more amino acids than any other form of chromium supplement.

Some interesting studies done in the UK have shown the benefit of chromium picolinate to soccer players undergoing weight training.

Those given 200 mcg chromium per day for six weeks gained an average of 1.7 lb more lean muscle weight than did controls, and lost 2.6 per cent more body fat. Larger men weighing over 75 kg (165 lb) did not benefit – possibly because they needed higher doses. Some sports nutritionists prescribe chromium picolinate supplements of between 200 and 800 mcg per day for athletes in training.

There is no evidence that trivalent chromium, the form found in food, is toxic. Hexavalent chromium or chromate (the type found on car bumpers) is highly toxic, however.

The richest known source of natural GTF is brewer's yeast, whose GTF is 10 times more active than that from any other food. Chromium-enriched yeast, with an even higher content of GTF, has now been developed.

- Dietary sources of chromium include:
  brewer's yeast
  black pepper
  thyme
  wheatgerm
  wholewheat bread
  meats
  cheese.

  NB Most refined carbohydrates have had their chromium content removed.

COPPER

Copper is essential in very small amounts for healthy functioning of many enzymes in the liver, brain and muscles. It is involved in the utilization of oxygen and in the production of adrenaline-like hormones.

Copper is also essential for the production of melanin pigment and for collagen synthesis, maintaining healthy bones, cartilage, hair and skin. Copper-containing enzymes are important antioxidants which either inhibit the production of free radicals or mop them up once they are formed.

- Desirable copper intakes are not yet agreed. Safe intakes for optimum health in men are thought to be 1.5–3 mg/day.
- UK average intake: 1.6 mg/day. Intakes range from 0.7–3.4 mg.
- Active athletes should aim for an intake of 2–3 mg per day.

Only 30 per cent of dietary copper is absorbed, as the presence of raw meat, excessive vitamin C, zinc and calcium in the intestines impairs bioavailability. The ideal ratio of dietary copper to zinc is 1:10.

- Foods rich in copper include:
  crustaceans
  shellfish
  nuts
  dried stone fruits
  dried peas or beans
  green vegetables.
- Plant copper levels vary depending on the copper content of the soil in which they were grown.

IODINE

Iodine is essential for the synthesis of thyroid hormones.

- EC/UK RDA: 150 mcg/day.
- US RDA: 150 mcg/day.
- Athletes may need more as they can lose up to 150 mcg per day in sweat.
- UK average intake: 237 mcg/day. Intakes range 100–420 mcg.
- Sports nutritionists prescribe iodine supplements containing

50–200 mcg per day for some athletes. These levels are not toxic, though supplements containing more than this may make acne worse.

Iodine deficiency is now rare in Western countries since the introduction of iodized salt. In parts of the world, however (e.g. central Brazil and the Himalayas) thyroid gland goitres due to iodine deficiency affect up to 90 per cent of the population.

- Foods rich in iodine include:
  marine fish
  seafood (e.g. shrimp, lobster)
  seaweeds
  iodized salt.
- In the UK, cow's milk is also a good source due to the iodization of cattle feed.

IRON

Iron is an essential element for the combustion of carbohydrate, fat and protein to produce energy. It also forms part of the haemoglobin molecule which carries oxygen in the blood, and myoglobin, which binds oxygen in muscles.

- EC/UK RDA: 14 mg/day.
- US RDA: 10 mg/day.
- UK average intake: 13.7 mg/day. This varies from 6.5–25.7 mg from food sources.
- Sports nutritionists sometimes prescribe iron supplements of 10–25 mg per day for athletes in training. More than this is liable to have side-effects, and iron is toxic in high doses.
- Foods rich in iron include:
  red meat
  poultry
  fish
  nuts
  wholemeal bread

361

cocoa
egg yolk
green vegetables
parsley.

- The form of iron (heme) that is most easily absorbed is in red meat. Non-heme iron from vegetables is up to 10 times less bioavailable. Overboiling vegetables decreases their iron availability even further.

Vitamin C increases the absorption of iron, while calcium and tannin-containing drinks (e.g. tea) decrease it. Iron supplements taken alone can also decrease the absorption of dietary zinc, manganese, chromium and selenium.

MANGANESE

Manganese is another important antioxidant that is a component of several enzymes protecting against free radical attack (see page 369). It is necessary for the synthesis of blood-clotting factors, cholesterol and the brain neurotransmitter dopamine. Research also suggests it is involved in glucose metabolism and the maintenance of normal bone structure.

- The optimal intake of manganese is unknown, but on average we excrete 4 mg manganese per day which needs to be replaced.
- US National Research Council suggested intake: 2–5 mg/day. Up to 10 mg/day is considered safe. There is no EC/UK RDA.
- Because of their higher metabolism of glucose and the increased mineralization of bone, athletes may need more than this. Some sports nutritionists prescribe supplements containing 2–5 mg manganese.
- UK average intake: 4.6 mg.day (half of this derived from tea). One cup of tea contains around 1 mg of manganese. American men, who tend to drink less tea, obtain an estimated 2.7 mg manganese per day.
- There is no evidence of toxicity – in fact, manganese is considered one of the least toxic minerals when taken orally.

If excess is consumed in the diet, absorption is low while excretion (via bile and kidneys) is high.

- Foods and drinks rich in manganese include:
  tea
  whole grains
  nuts
  fruits
  seeds
  yeast
  egg
  leafy, green vegetables/herbs – depending on the manganese content and acidity of the soil in which they were grown.
- Small amounts of manganese are obtained from meat, shellfish and milk.

SELENIUM

Selenium is another powerful antioxidant that works in conjunction with vitamin E to help protect against free radical attack. It is essential for cell growth and fighting infection.

- EC/UK RDA: 75 mcg/day.
- US National Research Council recommendation: 70 mcg/day.
- UK average intake: 65 mcg/day, with 50 per cent obtained from cereals. Meat and fish provide most of the rest.
- Athletes may need more as exercise generates free radicals. Excess selenium can be toxic. An upper safe limit of 450 mcg per day has been suggested for adult men. If supplements are used, they should contain between 50 and 400 mcg selenium and no more, unless prescribed under medical supervision. Additional vitamin E should also be taken. Interestingly, inorganic selenium (but not organic) is best taken separately from vitamin C as the latter may impair selenium absorption.
- Foods rich in selenium include:
  broccoli
  mushrooms

363

cabbage
radishes
onions
garlic
celery
fish
wholegrains
wheat germ
nuts
yeast. A selenium-enriched strain of organic yeast is now
commercially available.

In some countries, selenium deficiency is widespread. Lack of
selenium in the soil does not affect plant growth but causes a
muscle-wasting disease in grazing animals. In China, intakes of
selenium are less than 12 mcg per day, this lack of selenium has
been associated with an endemic weakness of heart muscle
(Keshan Disease) which is responsive to selenium supplementation.

In parts of the US, New Zealand and Finland, selenium is
added to fertilizers to increase population intakes. Average
selenium intakes among New Zealand men are 15–40 mcg per
day, although no selenium-responsive disease has so far been
identified.

ZINC

Zinc is another antioxidant mineral that is an important
co-factor for over a hundred enzymes. It is needed to switch on
certain genes in response to hormone signals. This initiates
synthesis of the specific protein that gene is responsible for
making; zinc therefore plays an important role in the sensitivity of tissues to hormones.

Zinc deficiency before puberty delays sexual development
and can result in smaller male sex organs. Deficiency in later
life leads to slowed muscle growth and impaired immunity to
disease. More severe deficiencies lead to loss of the sense of

taste, and muscle weakness.

- EC/UK RDA: 15 mg/day
- US National Research Council recommendation: 15 mg/day.
- UK average intake: 11.4 mg/day. Intakes range from 5.7–19 mg/day.
- Athletes need more zinc than sedentary men due to their higher fatty acid turnover, to replace zinc lost in sweat, and for the interaction of testosterone which helps initiate muscle growth. Some sports nutritionists prescribe supplements containing 15–50 mg zinc per day for athletes.
- It is worth knowing that taking any more than 10 mg zinc in one go can upset the stomach and cause nausea. Zinc seems safe at doses up to several hundred milligrams per day, but excess impairs copper metabolism.
- Foods rich in zinc include:
  oatmeal
  whole grain products
  yeast
  seafoods
  meat
  nuts
  milk
  eggs
  cheese.
  Moderate amounts of zinc are found in chicken and vegetables. In general, animal meat is a better source of bioavailable zinc than vegetables.

You can check your zinc levels by obtaining tests from a pharmacy. If your zinc levels are low, taking supplements of 10 mg zinc three times a day will cause a rapid improvement. If you find this level in zinc intake causes gastrointestinal symptoms, drop down to taking the supplement twice a day.

Soya products and foods rich in iron reduce the absorption of zinc from the digestive tract. They are best avoided within two hours of taking your zinc supplements.

Boron

Boron seems to be essential for the manufacture of some steroid hormones, especially those needed for optimal muscle growth.

- UK average intakes: 0.4–1.9 mg/day.
- Optimal intake: unknown. Suggestions of 2 mg/day have been made.
- Some sports nutritionists prescribe supplements containing 3–6 mg per day.
- Intakes above 50 mg per day may impair the metabolism of other nutrients.
- Foods rich in boron include fruits and vegetables, especially:
  soybeans
  peanuts
  almonds
  raisins
  prunes
  dates
- raw honey.

Claims that boron can increase testosterone levels and build muscle are misleading. They are based on studies in post-menopausal women – not in hefty young athletes. Increased testosterone levels would only be expected in men if gross boron deficiency prevented the body making its normal amount.

Molybdenum

Molybdenum is a co-factor for three enzymes, one of which is involved in the metabolism of alcohol.

- UK average intakes: 70–240 mcg/day.
- Optimal intake: unknown. Provisional recommended intakes are between 75 and 250 mcg per day. There is no evidence that

athletes need more than this.
- Intakes above 500 mcg (0.5 mg) cause the loss of excess urinary copper, while doses above 10 mg per day can trigger gout.

Molybdenum deficiency has been linked with a high incidence of oesophageal cancer in China.

21

ANTIOXIDANTS AND FREE RADICALS

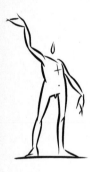

Antioxidants are protective substances that help to neutralize the damaging effects of oxidative reactions occurring within in our cells. The major dietary antioxidants are the vitamins A, C, E and betacarotene plus the minerals selenium, zinc, copper and manganese. They work by neutralizing damaging free radicals, either on their own or through incorporation into antioxidant enzymes.

WHAT ARE FREE RADICALS?

As in politics, a free radical is a highly unstable entity that races round picking fights and causing damage. The chemical version consists of a variety of molecular fragments which carry a negative electrical charge.

These unstable free radicals collide with other cell molecules until they achieve stability by neutralizing their charge – either through stealing a positive charge from another molecule or by off-loading their own negative one. This process is known as oxidation. It is estimated that every cell in our body is subjected to 10,000 free radical oxidations per day.

This is potentially serious as:

- Oxidized cholesterol is more likely to stick to artery walls and fur them up.
- Oxidized DNA can trigger gene mutations and cancers.
- Oxidization within the eye lens may trigger cataracts.
- Oxidized cell membranes and fats lead to premature wrinkling and skin ageing.
- It is estimated that 40 per cent of sperm damage is due to the harmful effects of free radicals. Oxidized DNA in sperm can lead to:
  - subfertility
  - developmental abnormalities in offspring
  - an increased risk of childhood cancers in offspring.

Free radicals are generated by our normal metabolic processes. Men with diabetes whose blood sugars are not tightly controlled generate twice as many free radicals as non-diabetic males. Smokers and others passively exposed to inhaled cigarette smoke or exhaust fumes also generate twice as many as their non-smoking peers.

Exposure to X-ray irradiation and to ultra-violet sunlight is a potent source of free radicals due to the energy in these waves activating and damaging cell molecules. This is one reason why both types of rays are linked with cancer. Other environmental agents that generate increased numbers of free radicals are the actions of alcohol and other drugs, especially antibiotics.

ANTIOXIDANTS

Antioxidants work by mopping up the negative charge on the free radicals without themselves becoming damaged. Their effects are summative and interlinked – for example, vitamin E that has mopped up a free radical is regenerated by a chemical interaction with vitamin C.

If we can keep our levels of antioxidants optimally high, most free radicals can be neutralized before they cause any

369

damage. That means ensuring an adequate dietary intake of vitamins C, E and betacarotene, and of the trace minerals selenium, zinc, copper and manganese.

Many experts now consider that reference nutrient intakes of antioxidant vitamins are inadequate. They were formulated to prevent deficiency diseases before the important antioxidant functions were understood.

The diets of thousands of people have been analysed and their dietary intakes of antioxidants compared with the subsequent incidence of coronary heart disease (CHD) and cancer. Researchers have found that those with the highest dietary antioxidant intakes have the lowest risk of developing these common killer diseases.

As a result of this work, the most protective intakes of antioxidant vitamins seem to be:

- Vitamin C: 100–250 mg/day
- Vitamin E: 30–80 mg/day
- Betacarotene: 15 mg/day.

Smokers and people with diabetes probably need to double these intakes. Various studies have found that:

- The risk of angina is three times higher in men with low intakes of vitamins E, C and betacarotene.
- The risk of CHD is reduced by up to 25 per cent in men taking vitamin E supplements for two years or more.
- Men with the highest intake of betacarotene have a 25 per cent lower risk of CHD.
- A high intake of vitamin C lowers the risk of CHD in men by 40 per cent – and the risk of dying from it by 35 per cent.
- High intakes of betacarotene also seem to protect against cancers of the mouth, throat, larynx, oesophagus, stomach, large bowel, bladder and lung.

Vitamins C, E and betacarotene plus the mineral zinc have their own separate and combined beneficial effects on sperm health (*see Chapters 19 and 20*). These effects are mostly due to their antioxidant properties.

Please send a stamped, self-addressed envelope if writing to an organization for information.

Contraception and Vasectomy

Marie Stopes
Marie Stopes House
108 Whitfield Street
London
W1P 6BE
Tel: 0171 388 0662 or 0171 388 2585
Advice and counselling on vasectomy, infertility, and sperm bank facilities.

British Pregnancy Advisory Service
Austy Manor
Wootton Wawen
Solihull
West Midlands
B95 6BX
Tel: (0564) 793225
Advice and counselling on vasectomy, infertility, and sperm bank facilities.

Family Planning Information Service
27–35 Mortimer St
London
W1N 7RJ
Tel: (071) 636 7866
Information on contraception and vasectomy.

Pregnancy Advisory Service
11–13 Charlotte St
London
W1P 1HD
Tel: (0171) 637 8962
Advice on contraception and vasectomy. Donor insemination service.

Vasectomy freephone
Tel: 0800 590 390
Twenty-two centres nationwide.

Infertility

Child
PO Box 154
Hounslow
Middlesex
TW5 0EZ
Tel: (0181) 992 5522
Advice and support to those having difficulty conceiving.

ISSUE–National Fertility Association
St George's Rectory
Tower St
Birmingham
B19 3RL
Tel: (0121) 359 4887
Information and support for infertile couples.

Sexual Counselling

British Association for Sexual and Marital Therapy
PO Box 63
Sheffield
S10 3TS
Information on therapists and clinics offering help for sexual and marital problems.

Impotence Information Centre
PO Box 1130
London
W3 0BB
Information about treatments and recent developments. Publications.

Identity Counselling Service
Marylebone Counselling Centre
17 Marylebone Road
London
NW1 5LT
Tel: (0171) 487 3797
Counselling for those with relationship or sexual-orientation problems. Fee charged.

Friend
86 Caledonian Road
London
N1 9ND
Tel: (0171) 837 2782 (Admin)
      (0171) 837 3337 (Helpline: 7.30–10 p.m.)
Counselling and support for gay men.

Gender Dysphoria Trust International
BM Box 7624
London
WC1N 3XX
Tel: (01323) 641100
Information and advice for those who are transsexual or think they might be.

Dr Sarah's Helplines
AIDS: 0891 336 349
Genital Herpes: 0891 336 303
Impotence: 0891 336302
Irritable Bowel Syndrome: 0891 336 300
Male Sex Drive: 0891 336 350
Orgasm: 0891 336 308
Penis Size: 0891 336 670
Piles: 0891 336 310
Premature Ejaculation: 0891 336 309
Prostate Problems: 0891 301 000
Calls cost 39p per minute cheap rate, 49p per minute at all other times.

Sexually Transmissible Diseases

Group B Hepatitis
Basement Flat
7A Fielding Road
London
W14 0LL
Tel: (0171) 244 6514
Information and support for those with Hepatitis B and their families. Leaflets, booklet, meetings.

Herpes Association
41 North Rd
London
N7 9DP

Tel: (0171) 609 9061 (Helpline)
Information and advice for sufferers.

National AIDS Helpline
Tel: (0800) 567123
Provides free, confidential information and advice on HIV and AIDS 24 hours a day, seven days a week.

Prostate Problems

Prostate Help Association
Langworth
Lincoln
LN3 5DF
Send SAE for information. Members receive regular newsletter.

Prostate Research Campaign UK
36 The Drive
Northwood
Middlesex
HA6 1HP
Tel: (01923) 824278
Information, visual aids, videos, booklets, magazine.

Better Prostate Healthline
Tel: (0891) 667788
Calls cost 36p per minute cheap rate; 48p per minute at all other times. Proceeds go to BLISS – Baby Life Support Systems.

Heart Disease

Healthwise Heartline
Tel: (0800) 858585 (Monday–Friday, midday–5 p.m.)
Information and advice on all aspects of heart disease, prevention and risk factors (e.g. high cholesterol levels, high blood pressure, diabetes).

Alcohol and Drugs

Alcohol Counselling and Prevention Services
34 Electric Lane
London
SW9 8JT
Tel: (0171) 737 3579
Help and advice for those worried about their drinking.
Leaflets; counselling.

Alcohol Concern
275 Grays Inn Road
London
WC1X 8QF
Tel: (0171) 833 3471
Factsheets, leaflets, telephone advice.

Alcoholics Anonymous
PO Box 1
Stonebow House
Stonebow
York YO1 2NJ
Tel: (01904) 644026
    (0171) 352 3001 (Advice line; 10 a.m.–10 p.m. daily)
Leaflets, newsletter, booklets.

Drugaid
1 Neville St
Cardiff
CF1 8LP
Tel: (01222) 383313 or (0800) 220794
24-hour help and information for users of drugs and their
families.

Drugcare
229 Upper Lattimore Rd
St Albans
AL1 3UE

Tel: (01727) 834539
Help and advice for anyone who sees drugs as a problem.

QUIT
102 Gloucester Place
London
W1H 3DA
Tel: (0171) 487 3000 (Smokers' Quitline; 9.30 a.m.–5.30 p.m.
daily)
Advice and counselling on giving up smoking.

Allergies

Allergy Support Group
Little Porters
64A Marchalls Drive
St Albans
Herts
Tel: (01727) 58705
Support for sufferers of any allergy.

Hair Loss

Hairline International
39 St John's Close
Knowle
West Midlands
B93 0NN
Tel: (01564) 782270
Information and support on all types of hair loss.

Back Pain

National Back Pain Association
31/33 Park Road
Teddington
Middlesex
TW11 0AB

Tel: (0181) 977 5474 or (0181) 977 5475
Leaflet, cassettes, meetings and general advice on back pain and back care.

Complementary Medicine

British Acupuncture Association and Register
34 Alderney Street
London
SW1V 4EU
Tel: (0171) 834 1012
Information leaflets, booklets, register of qualified practitioners.

British Herbal Medicine Association
Field House
Lye Hole Lane
Redhill
Bristol
BS18 7TB
Tel: (01934) 862994
Information leaflets, booklets, compendium, telephone advice.

British Homoeopathic Association
27A Devonshire Street
London
W1N 1RJ
Tel: (0171) 935 2163
Leaflets, referral to qualified homoeopathic doctors.

Council for Complementary and Alternative Medicine
Suite 1
19A Cavendish Square
London
W1M 9AD
Tel: (0171) 724 9103
Details on a variety of techniques and practices. Leaflets, booklets, newsletter.

Skin Problems

Acne Support Group
16 Dufour's Place
Broadwick Street
London
W1V 1FE
Tel: (0181) 743 2030
Help and advice for sufferers.

National Eczema Society
4 Tavistock Place
Tavistock Square
London
WC1H 9RA
Tel: (0171) 388 4097
Information and counselling for sufferers.

Stress

International Stress Management Association
The Priory Hospital
Priory lane
London
SW15 5JJ
Tel: (0181) 876 8261
Information on stress management and control. Leaflets, booklets, counselling.

Sleep

British Snoring and Sleep Association
The Steps
How Lane
Chipstead
Surrey
CR5 3LT
Tel: (01737) 557997
Information about snoring and sleep apnoea. Leaflets, booklets, newsletter.

Cancer

BACUP (British Association of Cancer United Patients)
3 Bath Place
Rivington St
London
EC2Y 3JR
Tel: (0800) 181199 (Freephone)
Information, advice and support for patients, family and friends. Leaflets, booklets, newsletter, counselling.

SHIP – Self Help In Pain
33 Kingsdown Park
Tankerton
Kent
CT5 2DT
Tel: (01227) 264677
Help and advice for all chronic pain suffers. Newsletter.

Well Man Screening

Marie Stopes
Marie Stopes House
108 Whitfield Street
London
W1P 6BE
Tel: 0171 388 0662
Tel: 0171 388 2585
Well man screening.

Barbican Medical
3 White Lyon Court
The Barbican
London
EC2Y 8EA
Tel: 0171 588 3146
Well man and executive health screening, fitness tests and cardiac exercise tolerance testing.